For the Love of Jugs

CRISSY FLORIO

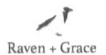

Raven + Grace

Contents

FOR THE LOVE OF JUGS

Disclaimer

I am not a doctor. This information is solely suggestive and informational. Please be sure to consult with your doctor, oncologist, naturopath, and/or functional medicine doctor before starting any new treatments or taking any supplements.

This book is not meant to be used to diagnose or treat any medical or psychological condition. The content of this book is solely for informational purposes only and is not intended to diagnose, treat, cure, or prevent any condition or disease.

You should consult a physician in matters relating to your health and particularly with respect to any symptoms that may require diagnosis or medical attention.

To My Pink Sisters,

This book is in honor of all my Pink Sisters—those who are fighting, those who will fight, and those we have heartbreakingly lost. This book was written solely with you in mind, with the hope that it will serve as a guiding light, a source of strength, and a reminder that you are never alone.

My intention is to do my part in making the path a little easier for future Breasties and, more than that, to empower you to tap into your own strength, your own resilience, and your own incredible power. You are warriors, survivors, and thrivers, and I honor each and every one of you. May you always feel supported, uplifted, and deeply seen.

From my heart to yours,

ONE LOVE
-Crissy

Introduction

It was March of 2012, when I finally completed my 200 hour yoga certification. Yoga's philosophy and learning a new perspective on living lit a spark within me, and I instantly saw life through a different lens.

When I was growing up, my mom was a nurse so meds and doctors were all I knew. However as I got older and was introduced to Eastern practices, I realized there was a whole other ideology of healing, living, and way of being from how I was taught within the concepts of the Western world.

Since then, I have dedicated my life to inspiring men and women to live their most authentic, healthiest, and happiest life by using my yoga teachings. Yoga has also taught me so much about myself, leaving me constantly craving the ultimate connection of self—Mind, Body, Heart, and Soul.

After my training certification, I continued to educate myself and adopted many practices to create a healthy lifestyle. I dove deeper and deeper into the holistic world and, naturally, lived my yoga on and off the mat. Some of my daily practices included yoga (obviously), meditation, Emotional Freedom Technique (EFT) tapping, journaling, and visualization, all of which I will talk about more in depth later in this book.

Life was great, I was a positive, strong woman, wife, sister, mother of two children, and friend to many beautiful souls. I was the ultimate model of a happy, healthy lifestyle—or so I thought!

On September 23, 2020, I was diagnosed with Stage Two Triple Positive Breast Cancer. I was ER positive, PR positive, and HER 2 positive with a tumor about six centimeters growing inside of me with another area of concern with calcifications. My world was rocked as you can imagine. Every fear-driven thought ran through my mind.

"How did this happen?"
"Why me?"
"How am I gonna beat this?"
"How am I gonna tell my kids and family?"

The list goes on and on. For those of you who have just been recently diagnosed or on the other side of the Big C, you know exactly what I am talking about. I crumbled at first.

When I first started my breast cancer journey, I was lost, confused, scared, and so overwhelmed; it all felt like a huge blur. Life was spinning, and I was a ball of emotions. I couldn't think straight, immediately became disconnected from my body, and so afraid to make the wrong decision. I mean my life depended on it, not too stressful at all (said no one ever)! :P

After that fearful day, the chaos continued with constant trips to the doctor for scans and tests. At the same time, I was constantly researching about the type of cancer I had and learning a new language (a.k.a., the cancer lingo), all of which kept me and my hubby busy. I went from someone who hardly went to the doctor or barely took medicine to someone who was going to have to put poison in her body to eradicate the cancer. That was a hard pill to swallow, pun intended, and I started to lose myself in the process.

Accepting the reality of my diagnosis, I immediately stopped working and teaching yoga, making health my first priority. I had to preserve my energy to get through this journey, and I knew it had to be spiritual, physical, energetic, and emotional. I had to heal it all to become cancer free!

I didn't think most doctors would agree or understand my request to integrate holistic healing alongside my treatments, but I knew, without a shadow of doubt, that I could not get through this journey without incorporating my yoga education to heal as a whole, not just in my breasts. So I let my intuition drive and proceeded to seek a holistic route alongside a journey of contemporary care. Thankfully with the help of my amazing husband and tribe, we ended up doing a lot of research together and cultivated a plan to merge the two and support my journey to becoming cancer free.

In the weeks and months to come, I completed six rounds of chemo (TCHP), one full year of Herceptin and Perjeta, opted for a double mastectomy with expanders, and eventually went in for round two of surgery for reconstruction. I decided to listen to my gut and graciously declined the suggestions to go through many rounds of radiation and take Tamoxifen. On the holistic side, I added pranic energy healing, meditation, white-light healing, grounding, and added the assistance of a naturopath, changed my diet, and added in more detoxification paths.

Naturally as a teacher, I want to share everything I've learned since my diagnosis to help my Pink Sisters create a calm, beautiful inner environment while you heal. Cue my why for writing this book. I am certainly no doctor, but my intention is to empower, inspire, and guide you, shining the light into the unknown darkness as you go through your journey.

We will take the woo-woo out of holistic healing and make it more mainstream, so you feel comfortable integrating and supporting yourself holistically while you go through your conventional protocol (if that is your journey).

Most people think it has to be one or the other. Why? Why does it have to be one or the other? Why not marry the two and get the best of both worlds? Knowledge is power, and the more you know, the better you are and the better you do. I have lived this journey and feel passionate about helping you to step into your own power and make decisions that feel right and aligned to you.

This book offers tips and suggestions to help answer your questions and inspire you to step out of your comfort zone by viewing this diagnosis from a different perspective. It is not written in a linear format but rather organized by subject. This allows you to move freely between chapters, depending on where you are in your journey. Whether you're undergoing chemotherapy, surgery, or radiation—or you're a Pink Sister who has completed treatment—you can easily find the information you need to create grace and ease along the way.

At the end of each chapter, you'll find blank pages for your personal use. Use them for journaling, note-taking, or as a space to write down mantras and affirmations.

This is your book, your bible, your guide, your workbook—whatever you want to call it!

I have also created something special just for my *For The Love of Jugs* Breasties. Please take a moment and head over to www.fortheloveofjugs.com to sign up and get exclusive access to your Breastie's Meditation Guide for recorded meditations that I created just for you. These recordings are specifically designed by chapter and topic to help you in your journey towards grace, ease, and inner power. Download the document and save it to your device or devices of choice. You will want to easily access them because as you can imagine, it is kinda hard to read and do the practices at the same time. Especially when I ask you to close your eyes. Unless you have some special power that I am unaware of! Ha ha!

Please know so much love has been poured into every page of this book, and hopefully you feel loved and supported while reading it. It was written from my heart, and I will be your biggest cheerleader, voice of reason, and breast friend. Every word is my truth, and I am cheering you on from afar.

You got this, my Warrior Sister. You Got This!

PS...
You may be wondering, *Why the title For The Love of Jugs?*
Funny you should ask. It's a great story! I was always a fairly little person with small, natural breasts and a sense of humor. Over the years, I learned to love my natural body and felt confident, beautiful, and sexy. Well, my brother-in-law, Mike, is a jokester and oddly enough nicknamed me Jugs a few years prior to my diagnosis. No hurt feelings on my end

because I was confident in my body, so I found it funny and went with it.

Needless to say when I was diagnosed, we decided to bring some levity and lightness to the situation, and my best friend started the campaign #OneloveforCrissysjugs. We had shirts, hats, bracelets, and even coffee mugs made for my tribe in support of my breast cancer journey. So as I sat down to think about the title of my book, only one thing came to mind: *For the Love of Jugs*.

This book will hopefully bring not only a sense of peace, ease, and grace into your journey but levity and lightness, too. Allow the laughs, giggles, or chuckles to come up along with any tears or frustrations as well. *For the Love of Jugs: A Breastie's Guide* invites you to feel it all. Enjoy.

ONE LOVE
-Crissy

Chapter One

Welcome to the C Club

AFFIRMATION:
I AM NOT CANCER, CANCER IS NOT ME.

"You have breast cancer." In a second, those four words change your world, inviting you into the one club that I can promise no one wants to be in—The C Club.

Numb and completely disassociated from your current reality, you feel as though you are in a dreamlike state, yet it's more like your worst nightmare. Every fearful thought will overcome your world, and you can barely see two feet in front of you, let alone see the other side of your cancer journey. In that moment, you feel as if life has been ripped to shreds and you are left lost, overwhelmed with five-thousand questions and no map to guide you. It's like you instantly freeze in time while life happens all around you.

Sound about right?

Don't worry I am pretty sure every cancer survivor, including myself, has experienced the same initial reaction. Even if you are the most upbeat, positive, optimistic person, those four words can rock your world and your nervous system in a heartbeat. While there is no exact timeline to shake the initial shock of a cancer diagnosis, it does fade as you come to terms accepting that this is a part of your story now. For some women, that may take days, weeks; and for others, it may take months, but at some point a glimmer of clarity does come back and you *can* gain a new sense of self and find peace in your journey.

But how?

Well you are reading this book, so you are already on the right track. I'm gonna share my secrets to creating a peaceful cancer journey to guide you to overcome this ugly disease with grace and ease, hopefully helping you create a deeper bond with yourself along the way.

* * *

In this first chapter, we are gonna go deep and set the foundation for your upcoming journey and healing process. I am going to be brutally honest with you. I mean we are Breasties now, so I trust you would be honest with me too.

This book will give you all the feels: we will cry, laugh, maybe provoke some screaming. I will ask you questions that may trigger you to get you to look at life through a different perspective. I may even say things you might not like, and that's okay, just be open-minded as you continue reading. Regardless, it's important to allow yourself to go with the flow as you read this book.

I know it's easy to lose yourself in your diagnosis between all the doctors appointments, research, and upcoming treatments, especially in the beginning. It's easy to want to hold on to the person you were before. It's easy to feel uprooted and not connected to anything.

> But what if I told you even in the midst of the scary diagnosis, you can shift from fear to peace in your journey, but you may need to make some changes to your thought process and your lifestyle?

How does that make you feel? Are you willing to create some change in your life? Does it sound unrealistic or does it empower you? I want you to feel empowered because you can do this! I am not saying it's necessarily easy to go through your cancer journey or to go through it with a sense of peace or grace. It's not a switch you can just turn on and BOOM, you are peaceful. No, no, no.

Grace and ease takes a conscious effort and self-compassion to create peace when staring in the eye of fear, especially with cancer.

> Here's the truth: Your diagnosis can either be a curse or it can be a gift. It's your choice.

It's all in how you look at it, and this truly goes for any traumatic experience in life. Truth of the matter is life is a gift, but oftentimes we do not see the importance of that gift until we experience a diagnosis, traumatic accident, or situation like this. Every year that we are on this planet is an opportunity to create a new chapter in the book of life. Some days and years are simply easier than others, but regardless, all should be celebrated and welcomed—even the most terrifying of ones like breast cancer.

I am here to inspire and encourage you to connect your Mind, Body, Heart, and Soul (MBHS) to heal through it. To change the narrative in your head, tap into your power, and fight for the life you are worthy of in order to appreciate the gift of life!

Sounds crazy, I know, and maybe completely unbelievable at this stage of the game, and that's okay. It will take some time to understand this view on cancer.

Just allow yourself the time to slow down, to connect, and to really listen to your body, so you can heal not only physically but spiritually as well. I invite you now to notice, how does it feel when you read that statement that your diagnosis can be either a curse or a gift? Clearly it's the gift you would return if you could and rather learn life's lessons another way, but nonetheless we know that is not possible.

Whatever you feel in this exact moment is totally okay; simply keep reading to further understand my thinking.

Repeat after me: I am not cancer, cancer is not me.

Repeat this affirmation three or four times or as many times as you need. You may even find yourself getting emotional saying it, especially if you haven't actually said it out loud yet, and that's okay too. Let the emotions roll. It shook me to the core the first hundred times I said, "I have breast cancer," because it made it feel so real.

Try to understand that the stress you feel at this moment is totally normal and almost inevitable, especially in the beginning of your journey. I think we can agree that stress can be a real bitch to our bodies, and possibly one of the many contributors to cancer growth based on some studies, so I feel this is a perfect time to offer you a meditation right now. You can't be open to receiving all the great information in this book to help set your foundation for healing if you are blocked, disconnected, stressed, and overwhelmed. Let's hit the reset button, shall we?

As I mentioned in the introduction, I have created a special Breastie's Meditation Guide with audio meditations based on topics throughout the book. All of the meditations and info I share will empower your healing, so if you haven't already, please head over to www.fortheloveofjugs.com to sign up for exclusive access. Put down the book and take the time to open up your meditation guide to listen to the Chapter 1 meditation. Once finished, meet me back here so we can continue our journey together.

Welcome back from your meditation. How do you feel? Observe to see if the layer of tension or stress has moved the sliding scale, even just a little. If not, then go through a few more rounds of breathing or bring back in your mantra—I am not cancer, cancer is not me. This is so powerful. Repeat this in your mind, or softly speak it into existence if your thoughts become louder than your breath. I invite you to be here now.

- Continue to repeat the affirmation out loud or silently in your mind, "I am not cancer, cancer is not me."
   - Let the breath guide you to be here in this present moment. Be right here, right now. Just breathe and give yourself some grace.
   - Bring your attention and awareness back to your breath and the moment.

Cancer is scary, no doubt about it. However, just know that this powerful tool of awareness and deep breathing, coupled with meditation and visualization, can help you shift from fight-or-flight response to calm and ease in an instant. I will talk more about that soon, but in this moment I hope you feel more calm, grounded, and clear-minded.

You will notice some extra blank pages at the end of this chapter, use the pages to write down any ahas, feels, notes, or journal about all that is coming up to the surface for you. This is your book and yours only, so please write whatever presents itself. If you do not have time right now to fully dive into your feelings, then at least write what they are and come back to this practice when you have more time.

Keep in mind breath-work or meditation will not take away your worries, but they can help to regulate your nervous system by slowing your heart rate, clearing your mind, and bringing you into the present moment, so you can make better decisions and see things a little clearer.

* * *

With that said, let's come back to the concept that your cancer diagnosis can be a curse or a gift. As I see it, you have two ways to process and take on your diagnosis. Let's see which scenario sounds more empowering to you.

1. As a woe is me, damsel in distress, powerless with a negative mentality, constantly looking outside yourself for answers, and clinging on for dear life to be the exact person you were before cancer.

OR

2. As a peaceful warrior with goddess or lioness vibes, ready to accept the challenge to fight for her life. I am not one to typically have a battle mentality or initiate war-like actions (Hello, yogi here) so I know it sounds like an oxymoron, but when I think of a peaceful warrior I think of power, strength, grace, and an undeniable sense of self compassion. Not the gladiator type of warrior, if that helps.

Which one sounds more empowering? Taking on this diagnosis like the damsel or the peaceful warrior? Ask yourself, which route feels like a better experience?

I pray you said number 2, and if you said number 1, this book might not be for you. The first scenario may come easier to some women because nothing changes, allowing them to try to hold on to the life they had before. This is a slippery slope that can make for a very hard, dark, fear-based road. When women choose to take that route, they hand over their power and go through life negative, unconscious, and stressed. All of which energetically creates DIS-ease in the body! More to come on this topic in the next chapter, but for now think of DIS-ease as another way to say "lack of ease".

Clearly what got you here wasn't working, so don't try to hold on to the person you were before. As the second scenario shows, a cancer diagnosis can empower you and give you the opportunity to take back your life without being a victim. It immediately elevates your power.

Again, we know you did not sign up for this, but each opportunity in life is given to us to teach us more about ourselves, allowing us to connect on a deeper level.

"Grow through what you go through" was a quote one of my friends told me at the beginning of my journey, and while I couldn't quite understand the impact of the quote at that exact moment, it did resonate with me, becoming an inspiration in my life. In order for you to *grow* through this experience, it's important to understand you need to open your eyes to a new way of being, thinking, and believing. And while you will never be exactly the same person you were before cancer, you can most definitely come out of this as a stronger, healthier, and a more conscious warrior than you ever thought possible. That, my Breastie, is a gift.

Living in the present moment and accepting your diagnosis is a huge first step. Saying you have cancer is a hard pill to swallow. I get it. I fully understand that it makes your future scary and the diagnosis real, but at the same time, denying it abdicates your power and hands it over to this evil disease.

Acceptance at its root is simply acknowledging all things, situations, relationships just as they are. The good, the bad, and the ugly.

Have you heard the saying, "It is what it is?" While some people may not like that statement, personally I love it because at the core of everything in life at this exact moment is how it is. At this moment, I have brown hair. The sun is yellow. You have cancer. All things are what they are at this very moment, because we are not attaching labels or meaning to them when we simply say it. It doesn't make it less real or less important, and it doesn't mean it all has to stay that way forever.

What's real is that life is constantly changing from moment to moment, and the real truth bomb here is that you, my friend, simply are a beautiful human being who happens to have DIS-ease in your body. Cancer cells are trying to take over, but you don't have to let cancer define you or steal your identity thus labeling you as some weak person. You are resilient and powerful beyond measure, and accepting your diagnosis will not change that. In fact, acceptance helps to create a stronger and more peaceful foundation towards your healing process. And so it is.

How to come to acceptance is different for everyone. What acceptance was for me will be different for you and for every other Pink Sister. Initially for me, it was understanding and coming to terms that life will look a little (or a lot) different from here on out.

In the beginning, I had to accept the fact that my life was going to take a different path than what I planned. As soon as I learned of my diagnosis, I went from working two part-time jobs, teaching yoga, and living a beautiful life to completely cutting ties with the world to focus solely on me and my journey. Not only did I need all my energy to process and heal, in order to get to the other side of this mountain, but going through my journey during the year of COVID-19 made life even more uncertain. I stopped teaching because I had no clue how my body and immune system would react and, quite honestly, I just could not give out my energy or inspire others.

I had to accept what was, so I could allow myself to process all the thoughts, emotions, and energy to shift from fear to peace in the situation. I had to accept quarantine life again, going back into my little hermit shell to shield myself from unwanted COVID-19 bacteria and germs and figure out my new life. If I wasted my time and energy on what I couldn't do, then I wouldn't have been able to see all the beauty that my cancer journey provided me.

Now I fully understand that everyone is different, and there are many women who have worked through their cancer journey because they either loved their job, financially had to, and/or working helped them feel normal and cope. I can honestly say I have no idea how my journey would be if I was not going through it during the COVID-19 pandemic and in an industry where I was constantly around people. It comes down to one thing...You do you, boo!

Don't ever compare yourself or your story with anyone else's. Do what feels right to you and your lifestyle, but give yourself some time and space to be alone with your thoughts and decide what's best for you.

Don't just try to go through the motions because that will only cause more issues down the road. Be honest with yourself during this process, because setting the stage for your fight is super important and also brings you one step closer to accepting your diagnosis.

* * *

Let's play a little game! Please take a moment and use the blank pages following this chapter to write down five positive words from the list below that you immediately connect with. Please, for the love, do not overthink it. Simply write down the words that jump out at you and give you all the feels.

Trust, Love, Peace, Power, Hope, Warrior, Happy, Heal, Determined, Strong, Calm, Compassion, Faith, Worthy, Grounded, Mindful, Grace, Support, Intuition, Ease, Fight, Confident, Courageous, Gratitude, Joy, Determination, Bravery, Respect, Introspection, Forgiveness, Acceptance, Powerful

All of the words above can be key attributes that promote peace and calm in the Mind, Body, Heart and Soul (MBHS).

Right now check in with yourself. How does your body feel when you read those words?

I know I immediately feel a shift towards a sense of ease when I read them. As you probably assume, you will have some not-so-great days throughout your journey, so I want you to have a powerful tool to quickly call on in the moments when you feel a little low.

Welcome to core values.

What is a core value? Core values are simply principles that may influence your behaviors, your thoughts, and your actions.

I believe your core values can basically remind you to keep yourself in alignment with your life's purpose, and in this case, your ability to go through your breast cancer journey with as much grace and ease as possible. I encourage you to use these in your journey as a tool or a practice to keep you (and your mind) present and positive. It is easy to stray away into a negative or stressed mindset at times, so use this exercise to encourage growth and promote mindfulness in your experience, guiding you to become a more in-tune woman than you were before cancer.

Once you pick the words (or the words pick you), write them down on the pages following this chapter. Below are a few questions to encourage you to dive deeper and journal your thoughts and feelings. Write whatever comes up for you, and keep in mind it does not have to make sense initially.

1. How do these words make me feel?

2.   Where can I incorporate my five core values in my journey?

3.   How can these words bring me comfort in the hard times and the good days?

4.   Where can these words help me create boundaries in my journey? Ie: family, work, relationships, etc.

5.   How can these words help me tap into my power and my intuition?

Next, I want you to create and write down an affirmation for each one to call on when needed. Use positive words and get creative; one or two sentences that empower you is all you need!

These affirmations and core values will serve as a reminder to be present accepting what is. Fill yourself with your own inspiration and love. Make them simple, so you can easily rehearse them in your mind and/or come back here to review when you need inspiration. You can also create index cards with your affirmations to use as a visual imprint or take a screenshot on your phone or tablet to look at them wherever and whenever.

The goal is to bring these core values and affirmations to the forefront of your mind to interrupt any fear, stress, or negativity that lowers your vibe.

If or when those moments arise, I want you to close your eyes, bring your hands to your heart, breathe in through the nose deeply and out of the nose, repeat the core value and/or affirmation in your mind.

Let it play on repeat in your mind over and over until you start to feel it in your body.

Then start to tap into the senses of the body to understand where you feel it in your body.

You can do this really anywhere, at any time. Just practice it any time your mind brings you into a state of fear or pulls you away from the present into the past or future. It's super important and powerful.

When I did this exercise, my words were: trust, mindfulness, intuition, love, and warrior, but I definitely found myself connecting with all of them.

For this exercise, I want you to just pick five because I do not want to overwhelm you. However, I do want you to have different ones to call on at any time for specific reasons. Each one can be powerful in their own way depending on the situation you experience at that moment—choose the one that feels most impactful and meaningful to you.

As an example, here are a few of my affirmations with my core values. I strongly encourage you to tap into your intuition and create your own that feel aligned and authentic to you.

Trust: I trust my body and surrender to what is.

Mindfulness: I live in the present moment to create peace within to heal. There is no time like now.

Intuition: I intuitively listen to my body to make aligned decisions. I am so powerful when I let my intuition lead.

Love: I fill my body with love and compassion as it is right now.

Warrior: I tap into my inner warrior to show up to my journey every day with strength, grace, peace, and ease. I got this.

Now you may think, *Come on, Crissy, that sounds easier said than done—can just repeating affirmations keep me from getting sad or angry? Can you really be positive and all peace, love, and happiness all the time?*

No, that's not realistic at all! The affirmations you create encourage you to live more mindfully, present, and with peace. I am not saying that you can just simply say a few positive words or have a positive mindset and Voila!, and it's all sunshine and butterflies every day.

Unfortunately you will have dark days, but if the good days outweigh the bad days, then you are winning in my eyes. Some days you may feel like yourself and others you may feel like lying in a puddle of tears. I wish I didn't have to say this, but everyone needs a good reminder to give yourself the freedom to feel all the feels! The good, the bad, and the ugly.

I had many days where I just simply felt angry thinking, *How is this my life?* or I felt sad not being able to visit with all my friends and family and cried alone in my room. It's okay; it's inevitable, so laugh, cry, scream, whatever.

> Do what you need to let yourself release the emotions because they are better out than in!

My yoga mentor used to always say, "The issues are in the tissues." It's so true; the emotions and the energy can oftentimes stay stuck in our cells if not released. Do not keep them pent up, but don't rush them either. Sit with them as long as you need to! There is no timeline or limit to how long you have to move through the emotions, and there is also no one *right* way to release emotions either. You can journal, go to a rage room, have a deep convo with a friend—whatever you need to acknowledge the emotions, feel the emotions, and then allow them to leave when fully expressed. Remind yourself this is like any other grieving process: Give yourself some grace and give yourself the gift of being present and accepting what is.

So far, Breastie, we have focused on:

- regulating your nervous system
- accepting your diagnosis
- creating your core values
- feeling your feelings

In alignment with all of the above, clearly your thoughts, words, and actions are just as important. What you think, say, and do can either make you feel super small and disempowered or help you to feel positive, confident, and strong.

Remember our first affirmation, "*I am not cancer, cancer is not me?*" That is a powerful affirmation in which you release the stronghold that a cancer diagnosis can present and not take on the power of it.

This may take some getting used to, but refrain from using "my" in the same sentence as cancer. For instance, when you say something like, "My cancer is in my right breast," you are simply owning the cancer as if you are cancer and cancer is you. It takes on the cancer label, which gives "it" so much power, nudging you towards feeling completely powerless and disassociated from your body. So a simple change from *my* to *the* is one little step towards a higher vibe such as, "The cancer is in my right breast."

* * *

On a similar topic, let's talk about your relationship with cancer and your language around it. If you talk about cancer or any of the cancer protocol in a fearful or negative way, it again gives it more power and substance while simply dragging you down into a low level, negative vibe. I will say my language with cancer has shifted since my diagnosis. At first, I felt I was going along with society's war-on-cancer tone. I said it all: I have to fight to kill the cancer. I am a Warrior! Fuck cancer!

The word cancer used to make me so angry, but then at one point, I realized that no longer served me. It didn't feel good when I said it; it felt negative and disempowering. But did I feel like a warrior? Yes, but as I mentioned above, we are peaceful warriors not gladiator warriors.

> We are strong, yet graceful. Sturdy, yet flexible. Grounded, yet hopeful. Fierce, yet loving. All of which can be felt during a cancer journey.

So, I decided to shift my tone and my language and try to no longer use phrases like kill the cancer, fuck cancer, cancer sucks, etc.

I also thought long and hard about how I used the word *fight.* Consider my perspective on this. You will see the word fight from time to time in this book. I am not asking you to fight against the cancer, because cancer cells are a part of you and a part of your body. If I said fight the cancer, then I would say to fight against yourself. That doesn't sound good to me.

Rather, I am asking you to fight for yourself and for your life. When I drilled down what it means to me to fight in a cancer diagnosis, I realized I see it as being your own advocate, being courageous, knowing your worth, knowing when to ask for help, knowing when to rest so your body can heal, and knowing that you deserve to tap into your power to get rid of the cancerous cells in your body and not feel like you are fighting against yourself. Consider it this way: It's more of a sense of standing up for yourself, which feels way more empowering when I put it in those terms rather than feeling like I am fighting myself or the cancer.

> The goal is to be stronger than the cancer, and your words and actions need to mimic that, so awareness is key.

Do you want the cancer gone? Hell yes, but let's consider bringing positive language into your journey from the start, which will help put your mind and body at ease.

As I mentioned, you will not always be peace signs and flowers; there will be moments where you fall off the peaceful wagon. That's okay. You are human, and you will get angry and probably throw a few F-bombs when talking about cancer. There are times when I still do, but they are few and far between now, which, again, lends itself to feeling more at peace and at ease. If you do find yourself in the position where your actions and words become negative and disempowering, it's important to be present and aware in those moments.

If/when you notice your words or your actions become negative or powerless, take a few moments to understand the why.

Where is it coming from and where in your body are you feeling it?

By noticing how it shows up in your body, you create more of a connection to your body and your nervous system. You owe it to your nervous system to hit the reset button, because no healing happens when you are in distress. Period, end of story.

Connect back to your conscious breathing, ground yourself in your moment, release the emotions, and, if you feel called, repeat your affirmations. You will start to feel the shift from fear to peace, once again putting you back in the driver's seat through your journey.

STORY TIME

I remember right before my first chemo, I was feeling nervous and angry about having to put "poison" in my body, and truly scared about it all. At that moment, my pranic energy healer, Faryl, gave me the absolute best advice.

She said, "You want to make peace with the chemo and cancer. You want to thank the chemo during your infusion so it guides you towards gratitude rather than fear. Say 'Thank you, chemo, go where you are needed and then leave the rest of my body unharmed.'"

That completely shifted my mindset from fear to empowerment and acceptance, helping to create a peaceful experience from that point on. I urge you to do the same, and start becoming more aware of your thoughts, actions, and the words you speak when talking about your journey. They can truly harm you or empower you.

Listen, it's no shock that cancer takes years to grow; it didn't just appear overnight. There could be many reasons as to why the cancer was expressed in your breast. You may never know the actual answer to that question, because it has been manifesting for some time with the perfect storm of stress, excess hormones, trauma, and toxins wreaking havoc in your body.

Similarly, your journey to peace will take some time too. Regardless, whether you are just starting your journey or you are a thriver looking to feel more connected and empowered about your life, give yourself the grace you deserve. Remember to regulate and live in the present moment, accept all that is, feel the feels, and affirm with positive thoughts and actions. Whenever you feel scared, dysregulated, or stressed, please remember your tools. Go back and listen to the meditation that I created or repeat your core values and affirmations to intervene and disrupt fear to create the shift towards ease.

> You are unbecoming your old self and becoming a newer, healthier, more mindful version of yourself, so take one day at a time, one foot in front of the other.

You are already well on your way to peace, my Breastie. Keep going!

AFFIRMATION:
I AM NOT CANCER, CANCER IS NOT ME.

Breastie's Notes, Thoughts, and Ahas

How can I remind myself daily that I am not defined by cancer?

What makes me feel strong and separate from this diagnosis?

Chapter Two

Healing as a Whole

AFFIRMATION:
I HEAL WHEN MY MIND, BODY, HEART, AND SOUL ARE
ONE AND IN HARMONY.

I had to think long and hard about how I wanted to approach this chapter, especially since I am not a medical doctor, doctor of osteopathic medicine, or a naturopath. I can, however, speak from my own personal experience and yoga background and encourage you to open your mind, seeing past the typical cancer protocol prescribed to so many Breasties before you.

You will find that with all the great information in this book, you get to decide how much or how little of the info shared feels aligned to you; then you can choose what you want to add or not add to your journey.

Here's the thing: There is power in choice, and you get to choose how you incorporate it into your own healing. My goal is to help you understand that there is more to your healing than medicine, surgery, and radiation. There are many practices that may help you experience grace, peace, and ease along the way. In my journey, I used both conventional and holistic medicines, which today continue to bring me such peace. I hope it does for you too.

With that said, this chapter will help you better understand why, in my eyes, adding holistic healing to your cancer journey is a game changer.

What is holistic healing?

Simply put, holistic medicine is the art and science of healing that addresses the whole person—body, mind, and spirit. It originated in Asia, so you may hear the term 'Eastern medicine' from time to time as well. The practice of Eastern/holistic medicine integrates conventional and alternative therapies to prevent and treat disease and, most importantly, to promote optimal health. Holistic healing is meant to inspire and empower you; it should not make you feel scared, overwhelmed, or intimidated because it is "woo-woo". (Personally I do not love that term, woo-woo, but I am sure you have heard the phrase when talking about holistic practices. Please for the love of jugs, can we get rid of that term woo-woo?!)

Many holistic practices have been around for hundreds, if not thousands, of years in certain cultures. It's one of the oldest medical systems. Thankfully, the United States, as well as some other countries, are slowly catching on to the powers of holistic healing. Maybe slower than I would like, but in order for holistic healing to become more mainstream around the globe, more research needs to be done.

Why? Because contemporary medicine relies primarily on research and science. In order for most hospitals and doctors to "believe" in natural or holistic healing, the research simply needs to be there. However, while there may not be a ton of research on holistic health just yet, especially within the cancer world, we simply should not deny the age-old techniques of Eastern medicine. I hope in years to come there will be more people on board and more research conducted to show the amazing power behind natural and/or holistic healing. I pray by then the term woo-woo will be brought to extinction. Or maybe we can come up with a better name?

Ha ha! Enough about that though. Let's continue on, shall we?

I feel it is my duty as a Breastie to share this information now because:

1. You will see the theme of holistic approaches throughout the book.
2. I want you to start your journey with an open mind and fresh perspective.
3. The Mind, Body, Heart, and Soul (MBHS) connection is (in my eyes) essential to your healing journey.

Let's first start with the Mind, Body, Heart, and Soul connection, which is fundamentally what I believe is the foundation of all holistic healing. It's the ultimate bond in creating harmony in your whole being. Notice I didn't just say mind-body connection like you may have seen elsewhere.

Let me explain. We know the first two, mind and body, are undeniably important and extremely powerful together because of their direct communication with one another. I am sure we have all heard, "The mind is a powerful tool."

It's so true! Think back to a moment in your life where you simply thought about something scary or negative and your body gets tense or freezes. Your mind tells you something is wrong and your body reacts by freezing. It's really the combination of the two that makes it so powerful, not just the mind. They constantly communicate with one another back and forth throughout the day. Your mind, a.k.a. your thoughts and/or emotions affect the body just as your body equally affects your thoughts and/or emotions.

We all need more connection to our body and the signals it gives us throughout the day. Heard of the "gut brain?" Have you ever felt butterflies in your stomach when you are nervous about a conversation or a presentation? That's the body telling the mind something is up and to be alert, activating the nervous system.

I could probably talk about this all day but will keep it short, because I know I can go down a rabbit hole and I will save that for another book. Ha ha!

Anyway, I love the power of the mind and body. I love how they speak to one another and help each other at certain times. I just want you to understand the importance of the mind-body connection and that it is not a one-way street. They talk to one another a gazillion times throughout the day.

While super important, the concept of just the mind and body feels incomplete to me. Adding heart and soul into the mix feels more balanced and whole. When I think of heart and soul, I immediately experience love and trust, which are just another couple of parts of the healing equation to guide you through your cancer journey.

Have you ever heard the saying, "The heart is the seat of the soul?"

Not sure where I first heard it, but wow, it struck me. When we add heart into the combo of healing and viewing our essence, it means we do all things from a loving, compassionate place.

> We know we are love and worthy of being loved as well. From that loving place, along with harmony in our mind and body, we are more open to accessing and trusting our soul, our higher self, God, or whatever higher power you believe.

Believing that my heart is the seat of my soul brings an element of loving compassion and a trusting, spiritual essence to accompany the strong mind-body connection.

I don't know about you, but that immediately sends me into a high-vibe frequency when I think about it. For me, it just confirms that when all is balanced together, the MBHS connection, we create a deeper level of unity, harmony, oneness, and faith—all driven by the power of love and connection as a whole, not just our bodies. It doesn't matter who or what you believe. Just believing that there is a higher presence by your side is sufficient. Marrying that with doing all things with love and compassion in your soul will help your healing.

* * *

With that said, let's circle back around to the affirmation at the top of this chapter: I heal when my Mind, Body, Heart, and Soul are one and in harmony.

Just writing that affirmation for this chapter not only felt like a warm hug to my soul but a direct line to that high-vibe feeling of connection and oneness. I know with all the craziness of the cancer diagnosis you may have lost that connection to yourself, and overwhelm may settle in and pull you away from feeling connected to your essence. This is why I am so passionate about encouraging you to think about your MBHS connection early on your road to healing and recovery. It's a valuable part of your overall holistic health.

The definition of holistic is:

1.   characterized by the belief that the parts of something are interconnected and can be explained only by reference to the whole
2.   characterized by the treatment of the whole person, taking into account mental and social factors, rather than just the symptoms of an illness

Notice the word 'whole' in both definitions? I believe holistic should have been spelled *wholistic*! You can maybe think of holistic healing as a secondary form of insurance to your contemporary medicine journey. Two is better than one in this case! This does not have to be a divorce where you pick either traditional Eastern medicine or contemporary Western medicine. Nope.

I promise that I will not tell you to pick one side or the other of medicine because there is room for both. You can use both methods together to support you on every level—physically, energetically, and emotionally. By adding in additional holistic healing practices along with your contemporary treatments, you consider healing your whole self and not just physically in your breast(s). That means you must also take into consideration your energy, your thoughts, your emotions, your food, your environment, your relationships and your past trauma. All of which fall under the MBHS connection in your healing.

With holistic healing, the root cause of the disease can most often be something energetic, mental, or emotional that is "stuck" subconsciously in the body. Contemporary medicine views the root cause as being the actual breast or where the cancer started. Sure chemo, surgery, and/or radiation might be able to physically remove the cancer, but what about your energy, your mindset, and your emotions?

The holistic approach takes all of that into consideration in your healing. You may never know the exact formula that contributed to the cancer growth, and I do not necessarily want you to stress or harp on the "Why or how did this happen to me?" because we clearly cannot go back in time.

Instead, I would love for you to be proactive about your current reality and incorporate some practices to help you release the energy, shift your mindset, and build a stronger sense of intuition, trusting this journey with your whole self not just relying on doctors. No amount of surgeons or medicine can strengthen your MBHS connection. Only YOU can! You have the power!

I don't know about you, but that makes me perk up automatically like, "Hell yeah, I got this!"

It empowers, inspires, and challenges me to want to form a deeper bond with myself, which then creates a sense of oneness deepening the MBHS connection. I hope this sparks a fire within you too and hopefully has you asking "what" or "how?" at this moment. The curiosity is totally normal, and I want you to hone into that curiosity as you continue reading.

> Trust me, and more importantly, trust yourself! You are whole, and you have the power within you to get through this with grace and ease if you start to shift your perspective just a wee bit. Follow along with an open mind, and you will find your way.

Before I list out some holistic practices, I want to talk about stress and circle back to the term DIS-ease. You may have picked up on this in chapter 1 and thought, *Is this a typo?* Nope, not a typo; DIS-ease is not meant to read as disease like you think and know it.

When I read the all too common word disease, I (and many in the holistic world) read it as DIS-ease, which has a whole different meaning. DIS-ease in this context means there is disruption of ease or even lack of ease somewhere in your body—mentally, physically, or energetically. It is important to understand that many diseases, such as cancer or heart disease, can only grow or form in environments that are not in homeostasis or fully at ease.

I say this not to upset you or to make you think you have done anything wrong. There are many factors or contributors in cancer growth, from environmental toxins, endocrine disruptors, inflammation to generational trauma or stress—some in your control and some not. Please do not add more stress to your life by thinking you did someone wrong. You have done nothing wrong! I mention this because it supports my mission and reasoning to help you open your mind moving forward, so you see the importance of healing through a holistic lens to create a harmonious life of ease.

Stress, also known as the silent killer, may be a huge contributor to creating DIS-ease in the body not only disrupting the MBHS connection but also your nervous system. All together can create a dysregulation of peace, ease, and homeostasis, which disrupts other systems of your body, such as your immune and circulatory systems. So many of us are in a constant state of chronic stress, but I want to be clear, you cannot heal your body and create peace in your body if your nervous system is functioning at a high level of chronic stress.

Let me repeat: You cannot heal your body experiencing chronic stress.

This is important to understand as you go along with your treatments and healing. Our bodies were designed to adapt to some stress. For instance, if a bear is chasing after you, your body will activate to tell you to hightail it out of there to keep you safe. Or when your body immediately reacts and pulls your hand away from a hot stove. In both examples, this is your nervous system activating the Sympathetic Nervous System (SNS), a.k.a. fight-or-flight. We need this fight-or-flight vibe to help us in certain times of our lives to kick into high gear and instinctively keep us safe.

The problem is most people constantly live this very intense, high level of stress, which keeps the body working overtime and activated. We clearly cannot function at this level all the time. Remember, we cannot heal when our bodies are constantly stressed.

This is where the Parasympathetic Nervous System (PNS) comes in. Your Parasympathetic Nervous System basically balances out the Sympathetic Nervous System with its rest-restore vibes. When the Parasympathetic Nervous System is activated, your body is calm, your heart rate slows down, your breath flows with ease, and your digestion is smooth. In this state, we conserve energy and create harmony within the systems of our bodies, so you can only imagine how we are more apt to heal in these conditions. This is where we need to live most of the time.

But how? I am glad you asked.

You can regulate your nervous system by reducing unnecessary stress in your life, creating a lifestyle of conscious awareness, and learning to love yourself and your MBHS.

Seems simple right? It is, but it isn't.

It takes a level of consciousness to recognize when we are stressed. That's the first part. Once you recognize stress, then you call on other holistic practices to help you shift towards ease.

For instance, remember that meditation from chapter 1? That was designed to create awareness, clear the mind, and calm the sympathetic response to activate your Parasympathetic Nervous System. I wanted you to experience the shift from fight-and-flight to rest-and-restore. Meditation is just one of many ways to support your nervous system to enhance the ultimate vibe of ease in your MBHS and is one of my favorite go-tos.

Listen, we all know that a cancer diagnosis is a disruptor to your peace, and your healing can be a long road if you let it consume you. Remember damsel or warrior? Damsel looks outside of herself for healing, but a warrior takes charge of her own life and steps into her power to heal.

Adding holistic healing to your journey is the warrior way to bring your body back to a state of peace, ease, and home-ostasis. Below you will find a list of many ways to calm your nervous system, heighten your level of awareness, and bring a sense of wholeness and harmony to your journey.

> Review the list to see which practices seem aligned and easy to embody. I am sure you have heard of some of these while others may be new to you, so do your research especially if there are any that make you go *hmmmm*. Circle the ones that seem most aligned and interesting to you.

Don't feel like you have to do all of them at once. Try one or two for about a month at a time because this could be overwhelming, especially if you are just starting out on this journey. There may be some you never try and that's okay, just see what calls to you. Be open minded and make sure you give it some time.

You might feel benefits immediately from practices like breath-work or simply changing your diet, while others like EFT tapping or white-light healing might take some time for you to notice a shift.

And as always, consult your doctor before incorporating new practices or therapies that could interfere with your treatment plan. For instance, supplements, acupuncture, coffee enemas, etc. may have to wait until you are done with active treatments, but practices such as meditation, movement, journaling, Qigong, etc. could be a few additions in your healing that you can incorporate now. Each one can help to nourish and balance the MBHS connection.

You may ask, *Will just one practice take the cancer away?* Probably not, and the goal is to help you start the shift towards a more peaceful, connected, healthier you on all levels, if you are open to it.

Many of these practices are more about a lifestyle change rather than reactive care so remind yourself: Any change is a step in the right direction towards your overall health and well being.

- Yoga (of course I had to put this first)
- Qigong
- Breath-work
- Lymphatic System Stimulation (consult your doctor if you had surgery and nodes removed)
- Exercise: low impact, strength training if you have the energy, cardio (just move)
- Meditation
- EFT Tapping
- Journaling
- Acupuncture
- Reiki
- Pranic Energy Healing
- Hypnosis

- Music Therapy or Sound Healing
- White Light Healing Meditations
- Inner Child Healing
- Vagus Nerve Activation
- Somatic Movement & Therapy
- Reflexology
- Chakra Healing
- Detoxification: castor oil packs, foot soaks, liver detox
- Salt Rooms
- Cold Plunge
- Hot Infrared Sauna
- Herbal Supplements
- Juicing
- Essential Oils
- Plant-based Diet

As you can see, there are many alternatives to incorporate balancing your MBHS. It's all about opening your mind to the possibilities, because when given the time and dedication, the design of our bodies as a whole is simply magnificent and so magical.

We have just been programmed to believe what we need is outside of us. I want you to know you have everything you need within you to heal on a deeper level if you believe in yourself and in your body. You are most powerful and healthy when your MBHS are one. Take a hold of your life; it's yours to live, so why not live it consciously with grace and ease? You gotta start somewhere—one day at a time, one foot in front of the other.

AFFIRMATION:
I HEAL WHEN MY MIND, BODY, HEART, AND SOUL ARE ONE AND IN HARMONY.

Breastie's Notes, Thoughts, and Ahas

What does harmony between my mind, body, heart, and soul look like?

How can I cultivate more moments of wholeness in my day-to-day life?

Chapter Three

Prep and Support

AFFIRMATION:
**I AM SURROUNDED BY LOVE AND AM SUPPORTED
EVERY STEP I TAKE.**

This chapter may be a little more straightforward with suggestions on how to physically prepare for the start of your treatments. From your team of doctors, to aligned support from friends and family, to preparing your home, there is a lot you can do to make sure you experience calm and ease while getting ready for all the treatments. I do believe these topics can be just as important as preparing your MBHS, because who you surround yourself with and the state of your condition matters. It can either help raise your energetic frequency or suck the life out of you right from the get-go. As Breasties, we know the latter is not the vibe we want, so keep reading and let's keep the high vibes going.

Create Your Team of Doctors

Let's first start with your team of doctors. I think it is important to surround yourself with a team who understands and honors your lifestyle and your beliefs. This goes for your breast surgeon, oncologist, radiologist, breast navigator, plastic surgeon, naturopath, breast cancer coach, etc. This also applies if you select a cancer center as a one-stop shop to help you navigate through your journey rather than individual doctors. Not all doctors and cancer centers are created equal, so ask around and read reviews from other local Pink Sisters to get a better understanding of their level of care and/or the technology they offer.

> As you explore options with your doctors, keep in mind this is your life we are talking about. Remember your power of choice, so if you feel anything less than the ultimate confidence in your team of doctors, your diagnosis, and/or the treatment plan, then ask around and get second or third opinions until you do.

Now obviously, time is of the essence because you want the cancer out of your body, but remember the cancer did not grow overnight. Take the time and do your due diligence to carefully select who cares for you. Think about not only who you want on your side but how open they are to adding some holistic practices to your journey and their approach to saying "buh bye" to the cancer. Some may offer surgery first, while another doctor could recommend chemotherapy first. It's kinda like the question, "Which came first: the chicken or the egg?" The order could be different based on either their schooling or your personal diagnosis. Regardless, every doctor will do things a little differently, so make sure you feel aligned and fully understand the treatment protocol before you get started. Listen to your body, a.k.a. your gut brain, in making your decisions, not just your mind.

You also should be assigned a breast navigator or breast coordinator to support you with understanding every aspect and angle of your breast cancer journey from appointments, to your team of doctors, cold capping, or even continuing support. Be sure to ask the cancer center or doctor to speak with the breast navigator sooner than later, as I have found they can also offer an immense sense of peace during this crazy time. My wonderful breast navigator was kind, patient, informative, supportive, and beyond accommodating throughout my entire journey...even still to this day.

Power of You and Aligned Choice

I want to take a moment to talk about the 'power of you' for a few. While I want you to feel connected to your team of medical support, absolutely no one's voice should be louder than your own intuition, especially when it comes to your life and making decisions.

> You are in charge of your life, not the cancer, not your doctors. YOU.

Many of us give away so much of our power to external factors that we lose the connection to our own intuition. Whether you are a spiritual being or not, the connection to self should be the strongest bond you share. You may have already noticed, but throughout this book, you will see words like alignment, intuition, essence, power, and other words with the same undertone. That is because I want you to be your own advocate throughout this whole process. I want you to make all decisions from a place of utter conviction with what feels right to you.

This is what I call an *aligned choice*. The concept of aligned choice gives you back the power in your life. Many people make decisions from fear or put so much trust in their doctors that they lose sight of what is right or wrong for them. They do it just because their doctors said so. I mean would you jump off a bridge because someone said so? No, probably not. Most likely in that moment, you would listen to your intuition, gut, or an inner voice to know that is not right, nor safe, and you would choose differently. Consider that same mindset when making any decisions in your breast cancer journey. Being completely aligned with your choices and decisions in your life matters.

Your voice matters! It's your life, so don't let anyone scare you into making a decision.

This is a perfect time for a quick break. I have created a meditation to help you tap into your power. Also known as your power source, your gut brain, your solar plexus, or third chakra. Please access your Breastie's Meditation Guide now to listen. And if you still have not gotten on board with the meditation, please go to www.fortheloveofjugs.com to get access. Listen to the Chapter 3 meditation. Please do not pass by this; this is a really empowering practice.

- ○ After your meditation, start to notice what difference you feel in your body.
- ○ Any changes or shifts in your physical, energetic, or mental/emotional state?
- ○ Do you feel stronger or more empowered in any sense?
- ○ Can you feel a shift from fear-driven thoughts towards your own power?

When you can re-align to your power, whether through meditation, visualization, or any other mindfulness practice, it gives you the opportunity to sense what feels right and what doesn't. It provides a moment of pause as an opportunity to shift and connect back to yourself—your whole self before making any decisions. To feel strong, aligned, and resilient—all of which are important as you go through your journey.

All decisions need to be made from that place of regulation and alignment to not only your intuition, but your inner power as well. Not fear! Always check in with yourself and make sure you are regulated and aligned.

Before making any decisions ask yourself, "Am I answering from an aligned place or out of fear?" Then listen to how the body responds for your answer.

Telling Friends and Family

As I said earlier, I am going to tell it like it is by being super honest, raw, and candid, so I would be lying if I didn't say that telling my children and family was one of the hardest things I have ever done. I literally have tears right now as I reflect back to the day I told them.

At that time, my son was a freshman at Florida State University (Go, Noles!), and my daughter was a sophomore in high school. I remember I could barely get the words out because it made it so real, but I had to become comfortable saying it because it was a part of my story.

I told them separately, and I was truly honest and emotional, not sugarcoating the situation. However, every word was backed with a positive tone in my voice. I did not want to scare them, but I did want them to understand the depth of what I was about to experience. And really what they were going to experience too. Even though I didn't know what it was going to look like, I knew they were going to most likely see me at my worst. I also wanted to assure them that I wasn't going down without a fight, and I was gonna tap into my inner warrior to fight this battle. I wanted them to see how strong I truly was.

I knew in my heart of hearts that I could not fight this alone so once my close family knew, I thought long and hard about who and how I was going to tell extended family and friends. I needed to gather my tribe so they could support me through it, even though I had no idea what to expect. I decided to create a private Facebook™ page dedicated to my journey. I called it Namastay Away from Cancer. I know, I know, it's kinda catchy.

I did this for a few reasons. I have a large family and lots of friends who were praying for me and supporting me from afar. I knew they felt helpless and wanted to be with me on my journey. I wanted them to know how I was doing and that their prayers and well wishes were welcomed to help lift me up and support me. Not to mention, creating this unified platform also minimized the constant texts and calls, giving me more time and space to heal through my journey.

Did I give every detail of my day-to-day experiences? Absolutely not. I gave just enough to let my peeps in, giving them updates on my healing. The page created a communication thread without me individually reaching out to every single person. It worked for me and my journey.

Clearly your experience will be different than mine, especially if you have little children and considering the depth of your relationship with your family. The point I will continue to scream at the top of my lungs is you have to do what you feel is right for you and your family.

Not only how you tell them, but also how much of your story you share with them is ultimately up to you. Regardless, I truly believe it is important for your closest people to know so they can support you and be with you along the way. I am not saying you have to tell the world or blast it on social media (obviously go for it if that's your cup of tea), but create a loving support crew to lift you up and help you as you embark on your journey. It could be one, three, or twenty-five people, and it doesn't have to be family, especially if your family dynamics aren't great.

Have you ever heard the saying, "Your vibe attracts your tribe?"

Having a supportive tribe is huge in your healing process in the upcoming months, as well as in any healing journey. You do not need to tell your negative, selfish aunt, Dottie, all the details for her to not lift you up and be there for you in the most positive way. (No, I do not have an aunt Dottie or any selfish aunts, but you get my drift Ha ha!). You set the tone for your healing and who you want by your side in your journey.

It can be friends, support groups, or maybe other cancer survivors who you've connected with who know what you are going through. Choose people who are positive, supportive, open-minded, unselfish, and honest with you. Carefully select a few you can trust and confide in, so you can be your most vulnerable and authentic self during this process. There are so many reasons why having a supportive tribe, community, and/or support system is beneficial to your cancer journey, but the one reason that sticks out the most is feeling connected. Being held and supported by loved ones is good for the soul and can do wonders for your healing—mentally, physically, energetically, and emotionally.

With that said, I also think it is important that you bring someone with you to all of your appointments if possible. A lot of information will be thrown at you, and there is no possible way you can receive it all. Not to mention, you may still be in shock, so having someone else there will provide two sets of ears and two minds at work to capture the information.

Release Expectations

I wasn't sure if I wanted to include this section, but I think it is only fair because my experience may cultivate a better sense of peace and acceptance in your experience. Around my third chemo infusion, I started to see more patterns of sadness, irritation, and frustration within me. They were different emotions than what I felt at the beginning of my journey. So I started to do a little spiritual digging to understand, *Why am I feeling this way?*

I realized it was regarding how people were communicating with me or their lack of. I realized that most people do not know how to communicate in these cases just like you may not have known how to verbalize what you needed in the beginning. The conversations I had were becoming less frequent and more invasive with people wanting in-depth details of how I was doing but only reached out every few weeks or months.

Not to mention, the one-liner, open-ended text, "How are you?" Whoa! That is a very big question that I felt deserved a call and got me thinking, *Do they really deserve the answer? Do they really want to hear about the many times I was back and forth to the bathroom, when I was sad, or how I couldn't eat because food tasted like concrete?*

What I realized was people want to help and support you, but they don't want to bother you too much at the same time, so they simply make themselves feel better with a generic text or reach out in a way that is easiest for them. I understand because I too have done that to let people know I am thinking about them but don't want to "bother" them. I realized that my expectations of others' actions ultimately led to my own disappointment. I know that expectations are the root of all disappointment, but I couldn't help the emotions when I was in it. They didn't know their actions had that effect on me.

The truth was I was lonely. I missed social interaction; I missed being with people; and I missed my normal life.

Within the loneliness I experienced, I was reminded of my yoga principles to let go of expectations. My expectations of how people would show up was neither right or fair to me or them, because they had no clue how I wanted to be supported, or how I needed them to communicate with me, or how I wanted so badly to feel normal.

If you do not communicate your needs, then how will they know?

As humans, when we expect others to show up a certain way, it can only lead to disappointment. Not to mention, adding the level of emotional stress and tension during a cancer journey just intensifies things. However, the combo of integrating good communication and releasing expectations can be a beautiful segway to deeper, more meaningful relationships. By doing this, you ultimately maintain peace within. Save yourself from this experience that I went through and take a moment right now to get real honest with yourself.

Close your eyes, take a few deep breaths, and start to visualize what support looks like to you. Ask yourself these questions:

- How does it feel?
- What emotions do I want to feel when being supported?

> ○   How can I communicate this with my tribe?
> ○   How do I want my tribe to communicate with me?

By going within and using visualization, you allow yourself to connect to all the feels in your body, mind, and emotions. This gives you a better vibe and vision of what support and communication authentically looks like to you. Then, and only then, should you verbalize it to your peeps with love, compassion, and understanding. Allow yourself to be present with what is, communicate your needs, and release the expectations over others. This truly sets the stage from the beginning, hopefully reducing frustration, and guides you one step closer to healing.

Take the Help and Support

Now let's take some of those visions and put into action how you want to be supported by your people. I know this can be super difficult especially if you are an, "I can do it all by myself" girl. I am not gonna lie; I am guilty of being that girl in the past. Trying to do everything myself, not loving to receive, and not wanting to burden anyone. Believe me when I say I know that asking for help can be difficult. And I know I am not the only one; there are a lot of women out there who feel the same.

Here's the thing, there are so many people who want to jump in as soon as they hear the news, so do not feel this is a burden on anyone. People want to help, so let them!

For me, in the beginning, it was a little overwhelming because I was spoiled with all types of baskets, gifts, and flowers from loved ones to prepare me for chemo. They showered me with well wishes and sent their love and support. It truly was so beyond generous and sweet, and I was taken back from the outpouring of love and gifts. I realized I was so overwhelmed because I have never been on the receiving end of so much love. I didn't ask for it and, to be quite honest, I had no idea how to receive it nor did I know how to use my words to ask for help at that time.

I simply didn't know how I wanted to be helped. I had never been in this situation before so how would I know? Right?

Thankfully, I had some pretty amazing people step up to make this all happen without me even knowing, which opened my eyes. As the chaos faded and the initial shock wore off, it gave me the time to get real honest with myself and remind myself, *It's okay to receive and ask for help when I need it most.*

Sometimes help looked like asking a friend to drop off a green smoothie, asking my mom to come down for my mastectomy, or calling my closest friends/family on my down days when I just needed to cry. It can also look like dinners, meal trains, rides to appointments, visits, crowdfunding services, gifts, or simply prayers. It is ultimately up to you to communicate how you want to be supported, so let your loved ones know what you need. People feel helpless, and these are simple ways they can help you.

It comes down to this: Take one day at a time. What you need to lift you up will be different from day to day, so give yourself some time to slow down and see what you need at that moment. Lean on your tribe to help you, to support you, to love you through this.

To piggyback off the support from your tribe, did you know there are also organizations that offer services for cancer patients in treatment? From cleaning your home to running errands to offering meals and integrative care. There are several non-profit organizations to assist you when in need, especially if you have no one to help you or financially cannot support yourself through your cancer journey. Ask your breast navigator, doctor, or research organizations in your area for more information.

Bottom line, don't struggle your way through your journey. Don't feel ashamed, weak, or less than; instead remind yourself that people want to help so put your pride aside and let them! You deserve it!

Creating Organization in the Chaos

There will be many times you may go through the motions of your journey unconsciously, which is what we are trying to shift, correct? I have one tip that can help: organization.

Being organized from the beginning can be essential in your cancer journey. Let's first start with the organization of all your paperwork. You don't want to miss any valuable information or misplace important documents so I recommend buying a folder and a journal/calendar in the beginning. Here's why:

1.   A dedicated folder is helpful because you will receive a ton of paperwork, prescriptions, and possibly want to take notes from conversations. Having a folder for your cancer journey helps you organize all the info in one place, making it easier to locate and review if/when needed. My husband titled ours (excuse the language) Fuck cancer folder. Ha ha! That thing went to every appointment with us because if we didn't know the answer to someone's question, then Voila! We had the paperwork to guide us.

2.   I also recommend purchasing a calendar and/or journal combo. You will have appointments out the wazoo, which can feel super overwhelming and you do not want to miss any appointments or calls. Personally, I used my calendar on my phone and loved the shared calendar feature to share my calendar with my husband to make sure we both were on the same page with all of my appointments.

I also found that jotting down the appointments on a paper calendar along with a space for journaling or notes was beneficial on a more intimate level. It allowed me to track what meds or supplements I took, how I was feeling that day, or track my energy levels, so I could look back for any correlations in my side-effects especially during chemo. I even recorded when I meditated, practiced yoga, and the days I exercised too. It came in handy when my doctor asked how I was doing, especially when the chemo brain blocked my memory (not sure if it is a real thing, but it felt real at the time).

Till this day I still have both my Fuck cancer folder and my journal just in case we need the information for anything, but once your treatments are complete, you could potentially burn it, which could be really cathartic too! Just be careful. Safety first.

Organization in Your Home

Before starting your treatment plan, take some time to prepare your house just like you will your MBHS. When there is clutter in your home, there may be clutter in your mind. Set aside some time to do laundry, clean sheets/bedding, purge, organize, and possibly prepare meals. I can promise this will make coming home from your treatments much sweeter, giving you more time to process and heal. Not to mention, if there is clutter in the home, there is most likely clutter in your thoughts and your energy too.

Remember you are trying to remove stressors in your life to create a peaceful healing environment, so you will want cleanliness, organization, and order within your house and in your body.

If you aren't up to cleaning and organizing then delegate, delegate, delegate! If funds allow, either hire a housekeeper for a few months or give lists of chores to family members and/or friends who can help you. Remember what I said before, don't be a hero; don't try to be a super woman—ask for help.

Create a Zen Space

Gift yourself the chance to create a calming environment somewhere in your house. I call mine my Zen Lounge (it's really only a corner in my bedroom but a zen space nonetheless). Call it whatever you like and make it your own. It can be a room, a corner, a closet, or a basement—doesn't have to be anything extravagant, just a dedicated space where you can chill to journal, be with your thoughts, express yourself, and/ or anything else you need to feel the feels in your healing. This should be a safe space solely for you, where your family knows it's off limits to congregate (unless you ask them to hang with you). It should bring a sense of comfort to help you grow through your experience. You want to personalize the area with the sole purpose of your peace in mind. Make it pretty, comfy, and calming by adding candles, crystals, inspiring quotes, etc. Ultimately, creating a positive yet healing vibe.

I will end with this because it is always worth the reminder. Remember you are in charge of your life; hone into that power and do your best to not let any other voice be louder than yours.

With intuitive power and some support, preparation, and organization, you can only enhance your healing experience. The more peace and ease you create in your home, relationships, and team of doctors will then ultimately reduce any unneeded stress in your MBHS during this time.

AFFIRMATION:
I AM SURROUNDED BY LOVE AND AM SUPPORTED
EVERY STEP I TAKE.

Breastie's Notes, Thoughts, and Ahas

Who are the people and resources I can rely on for love and support?

What steps can I take to feel more prepared and supported on this journey?

Chapter Four

Chemotherapy

AFFIRMATION:
MY BODY RECEIVES THE SUPPORT WHERE NEEDED
AND ALL ELSE IS UNHARMED.

As you are well aware, this is the Breastie's guide to creating grace and ease in your journey as a reflection of my own experience. With regards to chemotherapy, this is not a medical textbook going into detail of how chemo works or why one should or should not receive it. We can leave that for the doctors. However, this chapter will offer tips, suggestions, and recommendations that may help support you or someone you love if chemo is a part of your/their story.

Let's get right to it. The days before your first chemo infusion can be nerve-racking and overwhelming because, well, you have never done this before, and let's face it, the thought of chemotherapy can feel scary. Your mind may bounce from, *Will it hurt? to How will my body handle the side effects? to When will my hair fall out? to Is it killing the cancer or everything in my body?* etc.

It's safe to say you are not alone, whether it's potential hair loss, nausea, or weight loss or weight gain, all of the side effects can seem pretty damn intimidating. But as we have seen in many different examples, everyone is different and how chemo affects you will be different from anyone else you speak to.

The advice I give below may sound easier said than done, and I don't mean to seem insensitive, but here it goes...Don't overthink it. Just don't overthink it.

Crazy, I know, because all your mind wants to do is try to prepare you for survival for everything coming your way. To overthink is to immediately catapult you into the future. When you let your mind wander to all of the "what ifs," you are not present. You are instead thinking about what could happen in the future, therefore, creating a whole scenario in your mind that may never even occur.

Truth is you don't know how your body will adapt to the drugs and who knows? Hopefully, it will not be as bad as you think. Gift yourself the freedom of being present and surrendering to what is right now in this moment.

Remember this moment is the only place where life exists, *in this exact moment*. Try your best to stay here with me, especially as you continue reading. As I mentioned, this chapter is chock full of suggestions, inspiration, and tips to help you along in your chemotherapy journey, but I want you to remain as present and calm as possible. At any point if you start to feel anxious, I want you to come back to your tools of choice to help you realign from fear to presence. You can try breath-work, yoga, a walk, a chat with a friend, salt bath, or meditation to create presence in the present moment and be with what is rather than the mind conjuring up this whole story of 'what if?' We know that does not serve us well.

Now is a great time to take a moment and journal to release any of your fears if you are feeling overwhelmed.

Ask yourself: *What fear about my cancer journey is most present right now? If my fear had a shape or color, what would it look like? How can I visualize the fear softening or fading to reduce the overwhelm?*

Take a few moments to write down whatever comes up for you. Then once regulated, continue reading in preparation for chemotherapy.

Port Installation: Should you do it?

One of the first things that my doctor mentioned was installing a chemotherapy port, a.k.a. a port.

I was like, "A what?"

After researching the purpose of a port, I honestly was more scared of the port than the chemo initially. As I looked through pictures online, all my mind could see was them placing an alien in me. I kid you not! It looked weird, and the thought of the installation just freaked me out.

However, I knew it would be better than the alternative of getting an intravenous (IV) for each chemo infusion, and it truly was one of the best decisions I made. What I didn't realize in the beginning was there would be many more times I would need my port accessed than just the initial six infusions.

Follow me here: One poke the day of the infusion, one the next day to flush the port, then one more the following week to test my numbers and receive fluids, if needed. That's three times, every six weeks for my chemo cocktail, HTCP, not to mention if you continue immunotherapy once every three weeks for a whole year. Or for my Triple Negative girls, you may be going once per week for a while.

I honestly couldn't imagine having to get an IV in my arm every time, considering some nurses poke me numerous times before getting the one vein. My recommendation: Get the port. End of story.

Installing the port may be different from doctor to doctor. Some may put you fully under anesthesia to install the port, and some may do twilight anesthesia instead. For those of you who may not know what twilight anesthesia is, it is a type of sedation that numbs certain areas of the body, but you are not fully sedated. You are actually awake. Once again, I was a little freaked out about the thought of being "awake" during this but, honestly, I really didn't know what was going on at the time. I was talking with the nurses and doctors, listening to music, and felt no pain whatsoever.

Regardless of the route your doctor prefers, the port installation shouldn't hurt. However, it may initially look way worse than it feels. Mine was purple so it looked bruised, which could have also been the tape they put over it, but thankfully I didn't feel much. Even though it didn't hurt at all, I still did not like to touch it because it just felt weird to me. I learned to respect it as time went on.

You are stuck with it for a while, so rather than hate on it, learn to appreciate the little guy or girl. Ha ha! Maybe have some fun with it and name it. I didn't do that during my journey but see how fun that could be now! Paulie the Port, Patty Port, Pamela the Portastic Port...Wow, I am already having fun and wish I thought of this earlier. Ha ha!

One more thing about the port. Initially I thought I would want to cover up my port all the time, but oddly enough it was more comfortable uncovered than covered. I found myself wanting to wear shirts that didn't cover it rather than hiding it from the world. Regardless if you hide it or want to let it breathe, it's helpful to wear wide neck shirts or sweaters or button down shirts especially on infusion days so your port can be easily accessed. I hope all of this information gives you some comfort with your new friend.

Cold Capping

Another topic you may hear about or be interested in is cold capping. Not to scare you, but there are plenty of chemo drugs that can cause temporary or permanent hair loss, which is one of the side effects of the chemo cocktail I was prescribed.

I don't know about you but the word permanent was a little concerning, and I was scared my hair wouldn't grow back at all. Not to mention that my hubby (who happens to be bald) is amazing and took the reins to research cold capping for me. He told me that the bald look was his and his alone. I could not steal his "look"! I chuckled and didn't want to impede on his handsomeness, so I decided to add cold capping to my chemo regimen.

I highly suggest taking time to research to see if this is for you. We learned so much about cold capping prior to starting, but nothing quite prepares you for the experience of it until you do it. Below is some great information that might help you better understand the process and help your decision-making. Let's start with the basics.

What is cold capping?

In a nutshell, cold capping is a special cap designed to keep your noggin cold enough to constrict the hair follicles, reducing blood flow to the hair line so the drugs cannot make their way there. Ultimately, minimizing hair loss. Basically you wear a cap on chemo days for a few hours while you are receiving the infusion. The cap is approximately negative thirty degrees Celsius, which equates to negative twenty-two degrees Fahrenheit. (Yes, it's that cold.) The cap or caps are to be worn starting about fifty minutes prior to the start of the infusion of the drugs that can cause hair loss, during the infusion, and then for about two to four hours after the infusion. Typically, in total, around six hours.

On your off days, it's important to reduce the amount of heat exposure as it could damage your hair during this process. For months, you are encouraged to eliminate coloring your hair, not using a hot blow dryer or flat irons, not using hot water to wash your hair, limiting how many times you wash your hair, wearing hats on hot days, and using clean products with no parabens or sulfates. Basically, you do not want to get your scalp too hot or too overworked—not only during the chemo, but also extend it out a few months past your last chemo infusion. FYI: I did not cut or color my hair for four months after my last chemo infusion.

There are two different types of cold capping: Manual or automated, also known as scalp-cooling systems. Not all cancer facilities offer the scalp-cooling or cold-capping machines, so chat with your doctor or nurse navigator to get recommendations and/or to see if they have the machine in the infusion room or at a location close by.

My oncologist did not have the machine, so the manual option was the only way to go. As for what company to use, there are many companies to rent from such as Chemo Cold Capping, Penquin, Dignicap, and Paxman. You want to choose a company that specializes in cold capping with great customer service or one that provides everything you need in order to complete the process. We loved the company we used because we had the most wonderful representative to help us, and by us, I mean my hubby as he took on the responsibility of cold-capping extraordinaire like a champ. The company sent us everything we needed from the cooler down to the maxi pads that I put over my ears to eliminate any frostbite. Yes, you read that right. I wore maxi pads on my ears for six hours straight. Fun times.

Whichever company you choose should either have representatives to help you better understand the process and answer any questions and/or have great online tutorials to guide you. Cold capping can get kinda pricey, so select a company that sets you up for success. With that said, unfortunately, most insurance companies (if any) may not cover it so consider the cost in your decision making as well.

Side note about wigs: Really nice wigs are also pricey, but I have heard that some insurance companies may cover wigs, so weigh your options and ask for more information.

Manual Capping

With manual capping, there is no machine to feed the ice to your head, so you need another person to help you switch out the caps. I could not fathom doing that by yourself, so don't try to be a hero and please have someone help you. A lot goes into manual cold capping. You have to prep not only your hair but also your surrounding skin that could potentially have contact with the cap. Hence the maxi pads on my ears and foam on my forehead.

Plus, you don't just put on one cap and wear it for sixish hours. No, no, no. You must switch the caps every fifteen to twenty-five-ish minutes to maintain a certain degree of freezing on your head. You will also need to buy roughly eighty to one-hundred pounds of dry ice the day before each infusion (again another expense we did not take into consideration). Then, once you are done with your chemo treatments, you mail everything back to the company (i.e. the cooler, caps, gloves, and maybe a few other items). Don't worry though—you are not expected to send back the comb, maxi pads, or the foam.

Automatic Capping

Different from the manual option, there is the automatic or scalp-cooling option when the machine feeds the ice to the cap automatically. Even though your cancer center may already have the machines in their office, you will need to provide the actual cap and get it fitted for your head.

Unlike the manual process where you switch caps, in this option you only wear one cap the whole time with the machine. You keep the cap on the whole time rather than alternating the caps like I did. I do not know if there is a difference in cost between the two or if there are any other pre-setup measures to consider, so you may want to do some extra research.

> Truth bomb: I almost quit cold capping after the first infusion.

There is nothing easy about sitting with a freezing cap on your head for up to six hours with my hubby having to switch the caps every fifteen to twenty minutes. Just as I was about to get comfortable and in my meditative zone with one cap on, the countdown started over to get the current cap off and the new cap on. Then repeat for six hours. There was no time to fully rest.

While the first few moments are typically the hardest and coldest, I found the straps uncomfortable around my mouth and jaw. After the first infusion and inaugural cold-capping experience, I actually ached for days. I was going to give up. At that moment, I made the decision to go bald, but with the encouragement of my hubby and best friend, I decided to give it another go.

I created some workarounds with the straps and continued cold capping for all of the other infusions. I am truly glad I did. It was yet another layer of achievement in my journey. The discomfort of cold capping upon the discomfort of chemo was not easy, but I did it. I realized after each infusion that I can do hard things.

You too can do hard things.

I know I keep reiterating this statement, but you need to make the right decision for you. Cold capping is not for everyone—whether it's due to finances, no access, no additional help, or you simply want to be a bald badass—just make the decision that feels right and aligned to you.

Final Thoughts on Cold Capping

You will still shed some hair. I lost about fifteen to twenty percent of my hair. Thankfully I have thick hair so no one could really tell except for me and my closest loved ones. How much hair you lose depends on how well the cap is on during infusion, how well you care for your hair in between, and how healthy, strong, and amount of hair you have before treatments.

I don't want you to be shocked or alarmed by the clumps of hair that come out when you wash or brush your hair; it's natural. That's one of the reasons why we minimize brushing too much, washing too much, and exposing your hair to too much heat during chemo treatments.

I want you to be as prepared as possible with as much information to reduce any stress or doubts in your mind. Thankfully, my rep prepared me for this hair loss, and it helped minimize any freak outs, but I would be lying if I said I didn't have moments of tears when seeing my hair clumped in my hands.

Again, I am no doctor, but I want to be transparent. Some people may argue that cold capping may, in fact, reduce the chance of targeting any potential cancer cells near the hair-line. I am not sure if this is a myth or not, but I want to let you know so you can talk with your team of doctors about it. After hearing this, I still opted to do it because I felt it was the right choice for me. I felt as if the cancer was contained to my breast and nowhere else, but take what you want with this information. When in doubt, research.

Story Time

Let's end the topic of cold capping on a funny note. One night, as I was taking a shower before bed, I had a flash-back to when I would wash my hair during the cold-capping time period. Didn't feel comical then, but I can giggle about it now.

I absolutely love hot showers, well, anything hot really, I mean I am a native Floridian and I teach hot yoga, so clearly I love the heat. Needless to say, cold capping was an extra challenge for me.

Visualize this (well, maybe just from the head up). During that time, there was no way I could take entirely cold show-ers. As a compromise to save my hair, I would get in the shower and let the hot water run on my body, then when it was time for wetting my hair, I would turn it to cold, scooch out as far as I could to just let the water wet my hair then put the shampoo in, rinse, and turn it back to hot-hot-hot again. Then when ready, add the conditioner, let that sit for a while, then turn it to cold again, scooch out as far as I could to just rinse my hair, and back to hot-hot-hot water again.

I know, I know. Cold showers and cold water are good for us for many reasons, but whoa my body fights it big time.

Anywho, I just thought I would share the funny behind-the-scenes of cold capping from my own memory vault.

* * *

Prep Time

As I mentioned before, preparation and organization create more ease on every level, plain and simple. So preparing yourself for upcoming chemotherapy days should be no different.

I am sure you might be a bit overwhelmed with what to prepare, so low and behold, I have put together a list of tips, tricks, and suggestions to consider. Some of the products or practices you may need right away; some you may decide you need later in your journey; and some you may not need at all. This is just a list I have compiled from my own experience alongside some Pink Sisters who I had the pleasure of speaking with, so use your judgment and find what works best for you.

Don't Forget Your Teeth

Before starting chemo, schedule a dental cleaning and exam. Most oncologists will deter you from any dental work during your chemo treatment, so schedule a cleaning with your dentist before your treatments start. Main reason, if you have any cavities, chipped teeth, or loose crowns or fillings, you may want to have them fixed before chemo because they could get worse with chemo. Second, during chemo your immune system will be compromised, so it might not be smart to have tools and hands in your mouth just as a precaution-ary. You want to limit as much exposure to bacteria as possible to keep your immune system working to take care of the cancer. Make sense?

Also, it's a good reminder to continue to have a good daily dental routine during chemo. Depending on your chemo cocktail, you may experience dry mouth as a result of the chemo drugs. This sometimes can lead to plaque buildup, mouth sores, or inflammation in the mouth.

A dear friend of mine, and a dental hygienist, recommended that I really take care of my teeth and mouth during this time. I took her suggestions and did some of my own research too. I switched to a soft toothbrush for the time being, used a specific mouthwash along with Biotene to reduce the potential for these side effects, and reduced my intake of sugary and acidic foods. Seems to have worked well for me.

Hopefully you will not experience any major side effects, but hey, it doesn't hurt to have a good dental routine. Right?

Moral of story here: Schedule the appointment and ask your dentist about what mouthwash, toothpaste, or tooth-brush that can potentially help you during chemo. Keep those pearly whites happy and healthy.

Hydration Before During and After

You are going to hear me scream this from the top of my lungs multiple times.

Hydrate, hydrate, hydrate—before, during, and after your chemo infusions. Probably the most important thing you can do during chemo.

Dehydration can cause many issues and may increase some of the side effects like constipation and who's got time for that? And if you are on the other spectrum with diarrhea, then you definitely want to drink lots of water to make up for fluids lost.

So drink up. Even when you don't want to because your body is fighting hard.

You have been bombarded with meds, so keep drinking and flushing it out in order to help with your healing. It can be water, coconut water, or electrolytes (essential salts), but try to stay away from drinks with too much sugar. I have read many studies, listened to many podcasts, and seen many documentaries saying the same consensus that sugar does not necessarily feed cancer, like you may have heard. However, too much sugar spikes insulin levels, which, in turn, can feed cancer. I do think it is important to note that natural sugars, such as fruit, are acceptable because there are great benefits to certain natural sources of sugar. That could potentially be a whole other chapter, but for now we stay with hydration.

Get your fluid intake on. Period, end of story. No excuses. Your body will thank you.

On Chemo Days

Your chemo cocktail and whether or not you are cold capping will determine how long you visit your oncology office; therefore, how much stuff you should bring with you will depend.

Maybe buy yourself a cute chemo bag, tote, or backpack for chemo days, and fill it with items to ensure you have everything you desire to make your time there more pleasant. You will want to be as comfortable as possible and have things that make the time go faster. Take a look at the list below for ideas.

List o' Goodies:

- Chapstick to keep your puckers moist and plump.
- A charger for any devices such as phone, tablet, or laptop.
- A blanket or something to keep you warm and comfy. Personally, I loved my heated blanket, especially with the cold capping, but some may argue that heat is not good for neuropathy (a.k.a. nerve damage). I looked past that and took the risk.
- We can't forget about the tootsies. I loved warm and fuzzy socks. (I received so many funny cancer inspired socks—my faves were, "If you can read this, I am kicking cancer's ass."
- If you feel there is risk of neuropathy, then there are foot and hand covers for cooling the hands and feet to potentially reduce the risk.
- Peppermint or ginger candies and/or gum. Both are good to help reduce any potential nausea.
- Hydrate, hydrate, hydrate. Don't forget your cute cup and bring extra drinks.
- Food and snacks. You will be there a while, so might as well bring some healthy fuel such as trail mix, crackers, fruit, or peanut butter and jelly sandwiches to keep your energy up.

◦ A book, magazine, or cards. Bring something to keep you busy.

◦ A journal to record your experience, your thoughts, and your emotions.

◦ Download a movie or a few podcasts on your phone or tablet. If you decide to cold cap, it might be difficult to wear headphones or earbuds.

◦ Wear wide neck shirts/sweaters or button downs, so your port is easily accessible. It's usually cold in the infusion rooms, so long sleeves might be smart. Layers may be ideal if you experience hot flashes.

◦ Wear slip-on shoes to easily slip on for bathroom breaks.

◦ Probably one of my favorite gifts was an adorable heart pillow. It is a weighted pillow, and I would rest it on my belly or chest during chemo. It brought another layer of support and safety within. They come in different colors but, of course, I received the pink, which goes along with the breast cancer theme.

Here is the link to order if interested. https://a.co/d/dwyGkVT
(I am not affiliated with Amazon nor receive any perks from vendors listed in this book).

PS: Yes! I have created a *For the Love of Jugs* Chemotherapy Checklist for you to download or print. Head over to www.fortheloveofjugs.com or open your Breastie's Meditation Guide.

Now that you have all your items to keep you busy and more comfortable, keep in mind there will be men and women in the room getting their infusions too. You may want to spark up a convo with your chemo neighbor, and who knows, you may find a new friend or friends in the cancer world. Clearly, you have one thing in common.

I know I mentioned the importance of being supported by friends and family, but connecting with people going through a similar experience takes connection to a whole other level. Be open-minded to chat about your experience or personal life with others and listen to their stories, too. You may not only inspire others but also catch some nuggets of wisdom during your journey.

Besides conversing, making friends, reading, or watching shows, there are other ways you can ease your mind and pass the time while you receive the infusion. Remember my story about my pranic energy healer, Faryl? She helped me so much during chemo, but even if you do not hire a healer to support you energetically, you can do some energetic cleansing practices on your own.

You can incorporate some of the practices we already learned—like silently repeating your core value affirmations to redirect your mind and/or taking deep breaths to calm your nervous system.

The day of chemo can feel nerve-wracking and emotional, but with some preparation to create more ease in your mind and body, you can find some peace during your infusions.

Here is another one to add to your healing box o'goodies: white light healing. The universal symbol of white light is not only a sign for healing but can also increase positive energy, minimize stress, release fears, and enhance gratitude. I thought it was only fair that I create a beautiful white-light healing meditation along with some breath-work for you.

You know the drill, time to listen to the Chapter 4 meditation in your Breastie's Meditation Guide for the full experience.

Once you are finished with the meditation, I want you to say,

"Thank you, chemo. Thank you for doing your job to remove the cancer. Go where you are needed and leave the rest of my body unharmed."

Repeat this mantra and the white-light healing meditation as many times as you need.

Both can be especially powerful during the infusion and even the days after to continue to support the healing process energetically.

By doing this, you slowly shift from fear to gratitude. From denial to acceptance. From control to surrender. The vibration of the white light breaks up the tense cycle of stress to ignite healing, while the feeling of gratitude brings you into a state of peace. Both are very powerful together.

Now it's time to check-in with yourself after this practice. Tune into the body to notice how you feel.

Any difference in sensations from before starting?

Do you feel lighter? Warmer or cooler? More connected or supported?

No wrong answers here. I simply encourage you to invite a conscious and curious mindset to explore after the meditation. Regardless if it is a huge shift or a small one, a step closer to calm and peacefulness is the goal (write your thoughts here).

After Chemo

Now you are home, and I hope you are not sitting around waiting for side effects to kick in like a ticking time bomb.

Remember everyone is different, and you may or may not experience some symptoms that you "expect". This is the time to release expectations, be super connected to your body, and rest.

We will talk about side effects in just a moment, but here are suggestions to help your healing in the days to come immediately following chemo days. The goal is to create a calming environment internally and externally—in your body and in your life.

If possible, take a bath when you get home from your infusion even if it's later that night. Add some Epsom or table salt along with some essential oils and bubbles. You might even want to light a candle and make it a little self-healing ritual.

The warm bath will continue to encourage peace and calm, not only keeping your nervous system regulated, but also may aid in detoxification as well. If baths aren't your thing, then maybe a nice long shower where you can visualize the water washing away your worry. If it helps, you can also purchase a shower chair to make yourself more comfortable if/when you do not have much energy. Both options can be super healing and calming. Regardless, the idea is to create a healing ritual as a 'Thank you' to your body.

Try to get as much rest as you can. A good night's sleep can help you feel replenished and refreshed, but sometimes your sleep may be affected during treatment. Who knows why. It could be the chemo drugs or stress, but let your doctor know if your sleep is interrupted. They will have pharmaceutical options, but also talk to them about magnesium or melatonin if you would rather go the natural route. You need your rest, so do what you need for a good night's sleep. I will talk about this in another section, but medical marijuana may be a more natural way to help you sleep as well.

Eat what you can, and try to get some nutrients in you. At the end of the day, I was exhausted and not really hungry, but I knew I needed to nourish my body. I typically had some soup or something quick and healthy for infusion days. Something that was easy to heat up and warm, especially after cold capping. Soup was also good for my mouth and jaw, which typically hurt at the end of chemo days. Smoothies are another great choice if you don't mind the cold because you can add all kinds of healthy ingredients to refuel.

If possible, stay away from sodas, sugar, and highly processed foods unless that is all you can access at the moment. And, of course, continue hydrating! I won't go on another rant, but just another reminder of how important hydration is before, during, and after your chemo infusions.

Chemo Side Effects

Below is a list of some of the most common side effects associated with chemotherapy. While some may be self-explanatory, others might be less familiar. This list is here to provide you with a starting point.

It's important to remember that you may not experience all—or even any—of these side effects. The goal is to encourage you to tune into your body, understand what it needs, and know that there are supplements, medications, and other supportive options available to help minimize or manage the intensity of these effects.

Let your doctor know if you experience any of these so they can help you.

For instance for nerve pain, my doctor recommended I take a specific allergy pill to help with nerve pain. Yep, you read that right, an allergy pill for nerve pain. I thought it was interesting as well.

I don't necessarily love taking medicine, but it did help. Another thing I experienced was mouth sores, and my dear friend the dental hygienist recommended a specific mouthwash to help. There are workarounds for almost every side effect so, again, don't suffer through it. Other side-effects may include:

- Nausea
- Weakened Immune System
- Fatigue
- Constipation or Diarrhea
- Nerve Pain
- Brain Fog
- Mouth Sores
- Plaque Buildup
- Change of Taste
- Bruising or Bleeding
- Weight Changes
- Neuropathy
- Bloating
- Change in Skin
- Low Libido

- Mood Changes
- Hair Loss
- Chemo Brain

Also, here is something I did not know in the beginning: You may find that some of your side effects progressively get more intense or more common with each treatment. The chemo drugs accumulate with each infusion, thus your body may experience more intense effects due to this. Again, this is not to scare you as it may or may not be your situation. I just don't want you to be surprised. With that said, contact your medical team or doctor if you experience any of the following:

- A high fever, usually 100.5 degrees to 101 degrees Fahrenheit or greater
- Bleeding or unexplained bruising
- A rash
- An allergic reaction, such as swelling of the mouth or throat, severe itching, trouble swallowing
- Intense chills
- Pain or soreness at the chemo injection site or catheter/port site
- Unusual pain, including intense headaches
- Shortness of breath or trouble breathing (If you have trouble breathing, call 911 first).
- Long-lasting diarrhea or vomiting
- Bloody stool or blood in your urine

Side note: Before the start of each chemo infusion day, the nurses will check on your red blood count, white blood count, and your platelets. If too low, they may need to postpone your treatment.

Clearly that is the last thing you want, so here are a couple of tricks. You want to help your immune system so it works where needed (i.e. around the cancer):

1. Back to hydration. Make sure you hydrate yourself the days before your infusion.
2. Be sure to eat quality proteins and iron is important.
3. Either supplement or eat foods rich in vitamin B12, vitamin C, and folate.
4. Avoid raw foods if possible to avoid bacteria.

The night before my infusion days, I would cook a delicious piece of wild-caught salmon and broccoli to help with my blood levels. Thankfully, I did not have to postpone any treatments, and I pray you do not either.

Neuropathy (Nerve Damage)

Thankfully, I did not experience neuropathy, but I feel it deserves its own section because no one really spoke to me about it. Full disclosure, the information below comes from doing my own research with friends who have experienced it and my team of doctors.

Neuropathy is a potential side effect of chemotherapy that sometimes shows up after treatment has been completed. It is basically nerve damage that can cause tingling, numbness, or weakness in your extremities. There is no evidence yet as to why some experience it and some do not. Luck of the draw or perhaps the type of chemo drugs one receives may be the deciding factor.

Just know there are some things you can try to lessen your chances of experiencing this, or at a minimum, help lessen the intensity of it. Supplements, medication, or physical therapy are a few ways to help if you find yourself in this experience, but speak to your team of doctors for options to reduce your risk.

Exercise

I think by now almost everyone understands why exercise is good for us, regardless if this is currently in your daily routine or not. Yes, it is safe for you to exercise during chemo, and it can be especially good for you during your cancer journey. It may help reduce fatigue and stress, while improving lymphatic drainage, circulation, and your mood, which can all be super helpful in your healing through cancer. If in doubt, ask your doctor.

Don't worry I will not ask you to run a marathon daily or put yourself in some crazy advanced yoga shape, especially if you are a little shy or new to the exercise department.

But if that advanced level is the speed you were going before cancer, then hey, I say go for it, do what you can.

However, for most, I suggest adding or maintaining a simple exercise routine, especially during this time, because it can do wonders for your mind, body, and energy in your journey.

You may wonder, *Will I have the energy?*

Yes and no. There may be days you feel less than optimal, lessening your desire to move your body, and that's okay. On the flip-side, there may be days when you feel pretty good and energized to go for a walk, add gentle yoga stretching, or even lift light weights.

> Rule of thumb: Listen to your body (which you will see a lot in this book). If you feel kinda meh, rest might be best, but a slow walk outside could be just what the doctor ordered. Then on the days you feel more energized, you may feel up for a Pilates or yoga class or lifting some weights. Again, listen to your body and just do what you can when you can.

Supplements

There are a lot of supplements that may help with your chemo side effects, but I recommend talking to your doctor before adding anything into the mix. There are some doctors who do not want you taking vitamins or herbs during active treatment and some who may approve.

Regardless, there are many options to choose, but you want to ensure they do not negate or coincide with your chemo cocktail and your body will truly absorb the supplements. Not to mention that supplements can get costly, so another reason to understand what you take and why, so you don't waste a ton of money on something that will not help. Be sure all of your doctors are on board and understand what (if anything) you supplement during this time.

Changes in Taste Buds

You may have heard some women experiencing the 'metal mouth syndrome' or taste buds changing during chemo, which can sometimes be compared to a woman's taste buds changing during pregnancy. Different but kinda similar.

I did experience a change in my taste buds during chemo but definitely different from my pregnancies. At the start of my chemo journey, I remember trying to eat as many fruits and veggies as possible, but then my taste buds started to decline.

Around the fourth chemo treatment, it felt like a film was coating my mouth and everything I ate started to taste more like concrete or mud. This is different from the metal mouth I heard so much about. So keep in mind, you may have a similar or completely different experience.

At first it wasn't so bad, but it did become even more intense as my chemo treatments continued. Over time, I only wanted dry, dull foods like pasta or bagels. Even pizza at one point was no bueno, and if you know me, you know I love pizza.

By the last chemo infusion, I was down to broth. Nothing sounded good, but if a certain food sounded good, then usually the first bite made me think otherwise. This happened with many foods I used to love.

I don't share this to scare you or make you anxious. Instead, I want you to be aware so if it happens, you'll know it's a common and often temporary experience. Everyone's journey is unique—you may have a similar experience or something entirely different. Personally, my taste buds returned to normal about ten to fourteen days after my last infusion.

Along the way, you may need to experiment with different approaches to find what works best for you.

Here are a few suggestions to help eating during chemo:

- Do not eat foods you love just in case you create an aversion to them.
- Eat with plastic forks and spoons instead of metal.
- Drink, chew gum, or eat candy to help with bad tastes to hopefully reduce the taste in your mouth.
- Maintain good mouth hygiene.
- Try different marinades or seasonings if the food is too bland. (As you just read, bland foods were best for me).

Changes in Skin

My skin seemed to change a bit during chemo as well. It felt very dry, flaky, and my face was very puffy at times, especially just after infusions due to the steroids I had to take.

I mention this because it is so important what you put on your skin. Thick, very moisturizing products helped my skin, face, and body significantly. I don't think my skin looked too bad considering. Cleansing, toning, and moisturizing every day helped reduce the drab gray, dry look that chemo can sometimes create. Which leads me to this next statement that probably does not need to be said, but here we go...

The cleaner the products the better! No parabens, no sulfates, no fragrance, no harsh chemicals. That goes for beauty products but also house products, cookware, and clothing, just to name a few.

The more harmful ingredients you minimize right from the beginning, the better. Many of the products on the market have hidden toxic ingredients, one such as xenoestrogens, which are basically endocrine disruptors that mimic estrogen. If you have estrogen-driven cancer, then you will want to eliminate as much external estrogen as possible.

Simply making these changes may help more than you know, so do what you can. Don't go crazy throwing out everything you own; maybe change one product out at a time. Just food for thought.

Eyebrows and Eyelashes

There is a good chance you will lose some or all of your eyebrows and/or eyelashes. I lost both unfortunately; however, I made do with some workarounds.

I simply used eyebrow pencils and brow shapers to fill in what I lost, and it didn't look too bad if I do say so myself. Same for the eyelashes; I just used eyeliner to line my eyes so they didn't look so bare. The eyeliner at least darkened around my eyes, even though there were no actual lashes, so from afar you could hardly tell. I know some ladies get eyelash extensions or use magnetic lashes, but that all seemed like too much work for me.

Coming back to the theme of my life: You do you, Boo. Do what makes you happy, makes you feel beautiful, and what makes you feel most comfortable.

There are some really great serums and products that may encourage hair growth. Products like good ol' fashion castor oil to more fancy products like Grande lash serum to help with regrowth during this time. Find what best works for you.

I simply wanted a natural product I could use in a few different ways, so castor oil was the choice for me. To be honest, I am not sure how well or fast it worked, but my lashes and eyebrows are back for the most part. My eyebrows could be a little more full three years later, but that's okay—at least they grew back. I will take what I can get.

Now don't freak out, but some women may experience hair growth right after their treatments are over to only lose them again. I am not sure of the rhyme or reason, but I have heard of that happening to some Pink Sisters. If that does happen to you, simply go round two of what you did during treatment.

Low Libido

Unfortunately, chemo drugs (and some of the other medications after chemo) can interrupt your endocrine system and your sex drive. And let's state the obvious: You may just not feel your sexiest while going through treatment, which can most definitely add to the lack of intimacy.

Your body changes so, naturally, you may not feel like yourself at times, and this can be very difficult in one's sex life. I personally experienced low libido and have heard about it through other Pink Sisters as well. While sexual interactions might not be the same as before, that doesn't mean you have to nix them all together.

And keep in mind, this information is not limited to couples only. All of the information applies whether you are in a relationship or simply doing things solo.

First, dryness is one of the contributing factors that may make sexual interactions painful or unenjoyable. However, there are several products that can help create a healthy and pleasurable experience. Personally, coconut oil was my go-to, but you may want to research other products such as creams, ointments, or lubricants to help with dryness or pain.

Bear in mind that some may have estrogen in them, but from what I heard, it typically is not enough to make a difference and many women use them. Personally, for someone whose breast cancer was estrogen-driven, I was a "Hell No" to anything with estrogen, but that was me and my own decision.

Remember, in this book, we do what feels right and aligned to our own situations so You Do You, Boo! Do your own research and find what product works for you and keep in mind there is something that can help you.

Second, remember all the info above about exercise? Exercise can also influence your endocrine system and your sex drive by igniting hormones, such as testosterone, to spark your mojo once again. This is not the end-all-be-all but definitely can help.

I truly believe that having a regular exercise routine in your day to day, from the beginning, might even reduce the risk of low libido, or at least reduce the intensity of it compared to someone who is more sedentary. Do not get discouraged if you are just starting out moving your body because it still can help you—and hey, you gotta start somewhere, right? This is just another reminder to get your body moving to start bringing a sense of joy and harmony back into your life.

If you're in a relationship, open communication is essential during this journey. Personally, I had to find out the hard way that lack of sex drive was even a side effect. Thankfully, my husband was very understanding, as should all partners be.

Talk with your partner to nurture understanding and support between you. While discussing each other's needs may not instantly restore your libido, it can help cultivate patience, compassion, and emotional intimacy. This can be a challenging time for both of you, so be kind to yourselves, stay patient, and keep the lines of communication open.

In the meantime, you may want to also talk to your doctor because, in most cases, they may have some recommendations for you as well. Regardless, I know how vulnerable it is to openly talk about this topic—whether with your partner or your doctor; either way it is highly important in your journey.

Moral of the story: There are some actions and products that can help you in the bedroom. You just have to be willing and open-minded to some workarounds during treatment. While none of the above is an absolute guarantee to finding your spark again, I believe it's worth a shot! There are plenty of online support groups, therapists, pelvic floor, and sex specialists who provide resources and recommendations. Just consult with your doctor before starting anything.

Medical Marijuana

Okay, so I mentioned I would talk about this because it helped me during my chemo journey. I am fully aware that not all countries and some states in the United States are on board with medical marijuana, but I found it does help with side effects. If you are in an area where marijuana is legal (recreational or medicinal), it might be worth talking to your doctor about including it in your journey. They also may be able to even help get your medical card and recommend local medicinal dispensaries. But again, speak to your doctor about it or look into local medicinal dispensaries if you live in an area where it is legal to get more information.

Personally, it helped me with eating once my taste buds started to change around the second or third treatment. Medical marijuana also eased my nausea, and helped with pain, sleep, and relaxation.

I know some of you may not want to inhale actual smoke, which is totally understandable; however, there are many different ways you can use it medicinally. For instance, gummies, tinctures, and lotions are just a few options.

As we wrap up, hopefully you found valuable tips and suggestions to help give you a sense of peace and hope during your chemo journey. Just remember:

1. Don't stress out about the side effects that may never occur. Keep calm and go with the flow.
2. If you do experience side effects, try different things to find a sense of comfort.

3. Listen to your body and see what is best for you. What worked for someone else might not work for you and vice-versa.

I wish you well on your journey, and I'm cheering for you. You got this Pink Sister! You will be amazed what your body can handle; the human body is so resilient.

AFFIRMATION:
MY BODY RECEIVES THE SUPPORT WHERE NEEDED AND ALL ELSE IS UNHARMED.

Breastie's Notes, Thoughts, and Ahas

How can I visualize my body receiving the care it needs and protecting itself?

What practices help me stay calm and resilient during treatment?

Chapter Five

Prepping for Surgery

AFFIRMATION:
I OPEN MY MIND TO CHANGE
AND RELEASE CONTROL.

FYI: This section is primarily focused on mastectomies, but there is some valuable information for surgery in general. Even if you choose a lumpectomy, or are on the fence about surgery at all, take this information for what it's worth to you and your journey.

"Who cares, they are just boobs" was a common statement I heard from a lot of women when talking about surgery. Um, I don't know about you, but for me, I feel breasts are so feminine, beautiful, and sexy. Not to mention I breastfed my children, and there was that emotional tie as well.

I remember this time in my journey being a very emotional time. Maybe even way more emotional than chemo. You see,

I never wanted implants. I was always small chested, and as I got older, I learned to love and appreciate my natural body. I mean, you remember my Jugs nickname story, right?

It wasn't always that way. When I was in my early twenties, I felt a little self-conscious. Did I have moments where I wished I was bigger? Absolutely, but those moments never were stronger than the feeling of not wanting something foreign in my body. So you can imagine my thoughts when the doctor first mentioned the words double mastectomy with the option for reconstructive surgery.

We had to have this conversation multiple times—first at my diagnosis, then throughout chemo, and finally when the decision could no longer be postponed. The pressure of it all made me feel like I had no control over the outcome, as if I was being pushed toward implants I never truly wanted.

Could I have stayed flat? Sure, but I had to really weigh my options and make a decision that felt right to me.

So I want to start this chapter with the emotional piece of your surgical journey first, because regardless if you love the breasts you were born with or see this as an opportunity to enhance your physique, it will be emotional at some point.

Your doctors, most likely, will not be straightforward and open about it. As your Breastie, I feel you need to fully understand the levels of healing before, during, and after surgery. Then after the deep talk, we can get to the amazing list of suggestions, helping to prepare your mind and body for surgery too—I got you!

Making Decisions Prior to Surgery

You know I love to dig into the deep stuff first, so here we go.

Whether you were just diagnosed or going through chemo first, like me, emotional levels will fluctuate all throughout your journey. The truth is most Pink Sisters will endure surgery and make some hard decisions.

For some, it may be as simple as a lumpectomy or more involved like a single mastectomy versus double mastectomy. Then decisions like whether or not to stay flat, get implants, go right to reconstruction, or get the expanders first, then reconstruction. There are many options to select and some are more invasive than others. For instance, the Deep Inferior Epigastric Perforator (DIEP) is very involved.

As I have been singing from the rooftops, you have to choose which option is best for you. Personally, I opted for a bi-lateral mastectomy with expanders then reconstruction. While the implants were still a hard pill to swallow for me, being extremely flat or caved in, as my doctor mentioned, felt way harder to cope with than having foreign implants in my body.

I live in Florida where I am in a bathing suit, sports bra, or sundress probably eighty percent of the time so that was my deciding factor. It was a decision I made for myself and no one else, but it was not an easy decision. I looked at every scenario, got a couple of different opinions from reconstructive doctors, and ultimately decided from an aligned place. Just know this was my decision and mine alone.

Your decision should be based on your life, your beliefs, your body. Whatever your decision is, it's important to feel aligned and not worry about what anyone else says! It's your body and you have to feel good in it.

As I mentioned in this book many times, I believe there needs to be more talk around some of the emotions and our changing bodies. Quite honestly, I haven't met one woman who didn't feel like this was a major life-changing event, but I could be wrong—maybe there are some who feel that way.

I imagine those women are probably few and far between. It's a big deal for most of us, and we need to allow some time to adapt and grieve.

I went through many emotions during this time and some snuck up on me. The word grieving feels heavy to me; unfortunately, I have not found a word that has quite the same power, so let's continue with the thought of grieving, but maybe we can put a little spin on it.

I didn't grieve my old body like someone grieves a loved one, but the thought of my body changing and the uncertainty of it all did make me sad, nervous, and unsettled. There were a lot of tears and moments when I was in disbelief that this all was happening. With that said, I do not want you to discount your sadness if/when this comes up for you. Do not think you are a vain person if you get sad, angry, or anxious. You deserve to feel all of the feels and in the manner you need.

It doesn't matter if you still have your natural breasts or had enhancements prior to breast cancer, it is important to take a moment to honor and appreciate your body—both before and after surgery. While I did feel sadness at saying goodbye to my "old" breasts, it was equally important for me to honor their memory and embrace the "new." There's so much more to come on this topic.

Nipples

There probably aren't too many books that discuss nipples, but a breast cancer guide most definitely is one of them, so yes, of course, there is a whole section just about nipples in *For the Love of Jugs*.

I contemplated adding this section here (or in chapter 6) because we will discuss it later, but I felt there is room for some preparation here in the nipple department. As I am sure you know, there is a chance you may or may not have nipples when you wake up from surgery, which can be pretty emotional to say the least. The recurring theme of feeling overwhelmed with emotions and making decisions continues in your cancer journey. Regardless if you wake up in the 'no nipple' category or you already know that your surgery intends to remove your nipples, just know there are many factors that play a part in the doctor's decision to keep or remove your nipples. They will look at a few things such as current breast size, where the cancer is or was, and the perkiness of your current breasts. Details and logistics of medical procedures are clearly not my forte, but I will talk about emotions and tattoos when considering this topic. That I can help you with.

Removing the Nipples

If you know this is your route, there are some actions you can take prior to surgery to prepare yourself. Know that you have options after surgery.

First, have you ever heard of nipple tattoos? A dear friend of mine calls them 'tittoos'. So clever. There are tattoo artists who specialize in three-dimensional nipple tattoos to replicate real nipples. I have seen some, both in pictures and in real life, and Wow! simply amazing. They truly look like real nipples—it's insane. Take some time to research to see if anyone locally specializes in this skill. Obviously, this would be done well after your healing, if you consider this route but something to start thinking about now. Look at their work and talk to others who have had this done to understand the process of getting tattoos.

If you even think for a split moment that you might go down the tattoo route, then consider two things:

1.   If you like your natural nipples, take pictures of your nipples prior to surgery for tattoo inspiration. Even if you are not one-hundred percent sure if you want the tattoos, still take pictures so you have them in the future.

2.   If you don't love your current nipples, then guess what? Silver lining, you get to choose whatever nipples you want. Definitely a bright side to look at this situation. Maybe start researching nipples as you heal to get you inspired.

Second, you also may consider nipple reconstruction where the doctors reconstruct a new nipple out of your own breast skin. I thought it was interesting to hear that women will have a hard nipple at all times with this procedure. Some of you may like that and some may not so that's something to consider.

Third, if you choose nipple reconstruction, you may also want to consider an areola tattoo because the nipple reconstruction is just the nipple.

Regardless if you have tattoo nipples, reconstructed nipples, or get to keep your o.g. nipples, you may not have sensation in your breasts like you used to. This also may be emotional and is another great segway towards re-aligning.

> Remember you can't make aligned decisions or move towards healing from a clogged or emotionally drained space.

If you feel anxious with making decisions around your surgery, then it's time for your regulation practice. Do you remember how we regulated ourselves in the beginning of the book to grasp our diagnosis? You need to tune into the power of your Parasympathetic Nervous System, get grounded, and re-align yourself into the present state of being. This can be done every time you start to feel yourself getting pulled down into the tunnel of fear.

Before making any decisions regarding your surgery, take some time to regulate yourself. Open up your Breastie's Meditation Guide and practice any of the breath-work or meditations, and call to mind your core value affirmations, become present, and clear minded.

Shift from fear to empowerment. Then and only then can you start some of your research and decision making. You need to make sure you feel more clear, more open, and more calm rather than flustered, scared, or anxious.

Story Time

I remember about half-way through my chemo sessions I had a Magnetic Resonance Imaging (MRI) to see if the tumor was shrinking. And OMG was it ever—it went from about six centimeters to four millimeters in just three sessions, and I still had three to go! I was elated to know all that I endured with chemo was worth it!

However after he gave me the amazing results, my doctor started talking about surgery and reconstruction.

The thought of surgery and having to make decisions I didn't want to make led me into an immediate feeling of looming sadness and anxiety. I could feel my body freeze up, and as I got to my car, tears started streaming. I was sad because the surgery was real; it wasn't just talk anymore. I had to start making decisions like single or double mastectomy, flat or implants, then wondering will I have nipples or no nipples?

My mind started overthinking and getting overwhelmed again, which meant one thing: I wasn't present and fear was driving. I couldn't find the joy in the tumor shrinking. I couldn't celebrate how my body responded to the chemo treatments. I couldn't appreciate how important my spiritual healing was to this success, because I was blocked by fear and anxiety.

Clearly how my body responded was huge in my journey, but my mind immediately hit the fast-forward button big time.

Thankfully, in a short time, I recognized my lack of presence and realized this was not how I wanted to feel. I let myself work through the sadness. I had to feel the feelings before I could make any decisions. That lasted for a day or two, allowing my sadness the time it needed to process, to make its way up and out to heal that part of me.

Then I leaned into my spiritual tools to help me work through it. I did some meditations, journaling, and loving healing to bring me back to the present moment to find joy for what my body was doing to remove the cancer. I had to move from fear to peace with 'What is' in the moment.

Do you see how the theme continues? Fear will come up, out of nowhere sometimes, making your spiritual and healing practices all the more important to lean into for healing, especially when you recognize you are out of alignment from love, peace, and ease.

In that moment, I needed to honor all of the healing my body was doing in order to move forward and make decisions from a clear mind and not a fear-based mindset.

With regards to surgery, ask yourself while you are re-searching and making your decision, "How aligned am I in my decision making?"

I feel this is a great moment to bring up the topic of body image during your cancer journey. Clearly, surgery can be such a huge part of our bodies changing, but there are many reasons why your body image may change during a cancer diagnosis. Think about chemo and the hair loss, weight loss or weight gain, or changes in your nails. Now think about radiation and the changes in your skin like burns, redness, soreness, etc. I bring this up now, because I want you to be aware and notice if you start experiencing depression, anxiety, or disconnection from your body when thinking about surgery. If so, please fast-forward to Chapter 8 for some practices and information to help you shift from self-judgment to feeling more comfortable with your beautiful, changing body. Then, come back to this chapter and continue.

Preparation

Let's change gears from heavy stuff like decisions and emotions to some lighter topics around preparing for your upcoming surgical journey.

The more rested and comfortable you are after surgery the better for your healing, but it is important to start preparing before surgery. I am sure you have questions around how to prep prior to your surgery, so below are suggestions to help you prepare not only your body but your home and wardrobe too. This should ease your mind and make life a little easier on you. I incorporated things from my own journey, but there are some I wish I knew beforehand. But hey, it's okay. I get to share with you now so you don't have to learn the hard way. Here we go.

Request Help

Remember earlier in the book when you promised yourself that you will receive help and support? The days following your surgery will be hard to move around and be independent, so ask someone to help you—at least for a few days to a week following your surgery. Obviously your spouse may be your first go-to, but think about other loved ones, a friend you trust, or a nurse. You will need someone to help you with your drains, maybe washing or brushing your hair, and possibly with bringing you food, drinks, and medicine.

Lucky for me, my mom is a nurse so I asked her to come stay with us for the first few days. You see, my hubby doesn't love wounds, blood, or anything along those lines; and quite honestly, I wanted to give him a little break from having to take care of me, especially after a few months of chemo. It was great having my mom here not only to help with emptying the drains, but to keep me company in between naps as I healed. Sometimes it's the simplest things that you need so have your support ready on deck.

You also will not be able to drive for maybe six weeks or more after surgery, so try to do all your errands and grocery shopping before surgery. Right after surgery, you will have doctor's appointments for check-ups already lined up. With that in mind, ask someone to drive you to your appointments.

Also, if you have young kids, consider asking a friend to help with school drop-off and pick-ups. Think about their after-school schedule and activities, as well as making sure you have someone nearby to help. It's all about forward thinking, prepping, and scheduling, so planning this beforehand will relieve some stress and allow you to heal.

Exercise

Depending where your surgery falls (before or after chemo and/or radiation), exercise is an important factor before and after. While we know strong and flexible bodies are overall important in life, things like focusing on range of motion, lymphatic drainage, and simply moving the body for circulation are important in your healing, especially when talking specifically about mastectomies.

A sedentary body may do more harm by increasing the risk of lymphedema, infection, stiff joints, weight gain, depression, etc. Not to mention, our bodies are meant to move, and this is no different after surgery. However, I bring up the topic of exercise now so you can prepare your body before surgery, giving you a head-start in your training. Training your body beforehand will help your healing on all levels—mentally, physically, emotionally and energetically. Remember to get clearance from your doctor, especially if you do not exercise regularly.

You don't realize how much you use your arms to stand up from a sitting or lying down position. Or at least I didn't until I tried to get out of bed for the first time after my mastectomy.

Believe me, it becomes very clear the moment you try.

I remember I found myself trying to rock and roll like a ball just to sit up in bed. Thankfully maintaining a healthy and strong body before my diagnosis and during chemo helped me at this time.

I got two words for you: core and quads!

A strong core and strong legs can help you after surgery! Like I mentioned, getting out of bed or sitting down to use the bathroom may be a challenge if you have a weak body and can't use your arms. So use this as a reminder to learn to love chair pose and get those squats on to strengthen your legs. And don't forget those planks and Pilates exercises to tap into your core.

Head over to www.fortheloveofjugs.com for some tutorials and videos to help you. I have also included some simple yoga postures and Pilates exercises to incorporate into your daily routine leading up to your surgery.

Becoming stronger and more flexible in those areas can be an added bonus to help you feel better, heal faster, and have more energy. This will also help you to once again feel empowered about your body. Please do it sooner than later (if your energy allows), giving your body a head start before surgery.

Range of motion is also something to think about before and after surgery. Depending on what type of surgery you choose, it may hinder your range of motion on one or both sides, especially in the shoulder and chest region.

While my team brought up the idea of Physical Therapy (PT) beforehand, the importance of making it necessary before or after was never really emphasized (probably because of my yoga background). I do wish I made PT part of my journey. Personally I was really nervous and a little unclear as to what I should do or not do after surgery, regardless of my yoga knowledge of the body.

I was in pain and afraid to move the wrong way to potentially interfere with the stitches and the great work my plastic surgeon did. I think it would have been super helpful to know and understand what exercises to do and which to avoid. I used my best judgment and think I did a great job, because I only have a little weakness and minimal limitation in my range of motion on the side where the cancer was.

Not too bad, but again I want you to prepare as much as possible before, during, and after. Ask your team of doctors to either give you some exercises to do before and after and/ or refer you to a great PT who specializes in breast reconstruction.

Another great way to prep your body is to start walking. Outside or on a treadmill, it doesn't matter, just get moving. Walking helps our lymphatic system, cardiovascular system, immune system, and other important functions. It also helps clear your mind when you can either put on some music or podcast, or simply connect to the sounds of nature to get out of your mind! It may also help to relieve some of the muscle tightness and achiness too, so that's a bonus.

By starting your walking routine before surgery, you will help build your endurance to begin again shortly after your surgery. You may walk a little slower, and that's okay; anything is better than just laying around in bed.

Prepare and Organize Your Home

As I mentioned earlier, preparation and organization are key in many aspects, but within your home prior to surgery can be of the utmost importance. Remember, if there's chaos in your home, there is chaos in the mind and body. If your house is cluttered, messy, or unorganized, it can make for a hard recovery.

I promise you organization and preparation will make life a little easier. You will not be able to vacuum or do many house chores that involve using your arms or heavy lifting for some time, so prep your home by doing chores beforehand or delegating house chores, so it's one less thing to think about. Here are a few additional suggestions:

1. Think about what dishes, pots, pans, coffee mugs, spices, etc. that you use on a regular basis that currently may be higher up in your cabinets. You will not be able to lift your arms after the surgery. What items can you place on the counter for the time being? Organize one corner or a part of the counter that you can keep those most-used items to grab easily, because there will be a time when you want to start being a little more independent after surgery. You will be much happier if you don't need to ask your partner, spouse, or child to get the coffee mug down.

2.   No lifting heavy objects. Think about what products in your home are heavy and split them into smaller containers so they are easier to lift.

3.   You most likely will not feel like cooking. At a minimum for the first few days—personally I didn't want to cook for weeks Ha ha! You could either think about meal prepping to fill your fridge and/or freezer with yummy, healthy, and easy-to-heat-up meals prior to your surgery, if you are up to it. Or this may be a good time to ask a friend for a meal train. That way, meals can be delivered for at least the first couple of weeks to take some load off of your family while you heal. Don't forget to specify what you like and don't like, so you do not end up with a Shepherd's Pie or meatloaf if you don't eat meat. You get my drift? You can even ask for gift cards for your favorite local restaurants to simply order in.

4.   Laying down flat will not work after surgery. You will need to sleep upright for a few weeks, so purchasing or renting a recliner from a medical supply store would be wise. I don't believe those are too expensive. Now this may be a little out of your budget, but here's a suggestion that helped me. You can consider purchasing an adjustable bed (or maybe you already have one). Thankfully, my hubby and I bought one in 2019, not knowing that it would be a lifesaver in my healing. I basically slept upright for six to eight weeks, and my hubby had to sleep in another room for a few weeks because there was no way he was sleeping upright too. But that's okay. I know he loves me and would do anything for me, but the boy needs his sleep. Circling back

to bed or recliner, whatever you choose, just make sure it is comfortable because you need your sleep to heal and it will take a few weeks.

5.   Think about times you may want to sleep in or take a nap while healing. With that in mind, try to find the perfect healing spot to put your recliner where you won't be interrupted with the family watching TV or making breakfast. Then, set up the space with your recliner or bed and include an accessible side table to hold your water, meds, healing crystals, books, etc. Make it peaceful and try to keep everything at a short arm's distance.

6.   You will not be able to get your breasts wet as long as you have the drains in, so this may disrupt, for a short time, how you normally bathe or shower. The bathtub was great for me. I just filled up the tub to my belly button and was able to bathe without the fear of getting my breasts, incision sites, or drains wet. If you do not have a bathtub, you may want to do a sponge bath, or you can temporarily switch out your shower head to a handheld one to make showering easier. The goal is not to get the incision or the drains wet.

7.   A small collapsible lap or tray table might come in handy for eating, journaling, or a place to hold your tablet or computer during your healing. A friend of mine bought one for me before chemo and it really came in handy. I am using it as I type this very sentence.

8.   Another item I loved was a mastectomy pillow. I actually used this in the car more than I did sleeping because it provided the seat-belt a place to rest extended

out instead of on my chest, which was tender. Be sure to pack it for the hospital so you have it in your car after surgery. You can thank me later.

I also used it a lot when sitting on the couch, which gave me a sense of comfort and a place to put my arms, which also felt very protective, especially around pets or young children. And yes, there were times I used it in bed too; it was a staple piece during my surgery recovery.

9.　Both anesthesia and pain meds can sometimes enhance the risk of constipation after a surgery, so it is important to take that into consideration before the day of your surgery. There are many ways you can naturally help to reduce constipation, such as increasing your fiber intake with diet and hydration. Leafy greens, chia seeds, prunes, lentils, or beans are great for fiber. You can also have stool softeners or laxatives available after surgery if needed.

Your Breast Cancer Surgery Wardrobe

Moving on to your breast cancer surgery wardrobe. What you put on your body after the surgery, as far as your clothes goes, can be tricky. You will need to consider your pajamas, shirts, shoes, and bras as you heal. You will have limited range, strength, and use of your arms, so you will not be able to raise them overhead, behind you, or be able to pull clothes up.

Not to mention, for the first few weeks, you may also have drains if you have a single or double mastectomy and they can get in the way. Don't worry, they sound scarier than they are, and I will discuss more about drains in the next chapter. For now, here are some ideas for your closet that you can purchase prior to the surgery to make life a little easier.

1. Compression bras. Honestly you will want supportive bras—you will feel more comfortable with your boobies locked, loaded, and held in tight. Most likely your hospital or surgery center will send you home with a compression garment, but you still might want to purchase some of your own. Get ones with a zipper in front, not clasping in back, because you will not be able to reach around your back to clasp. Nor will you want to wear bras that you have to pull up or that are designed to be put on overhead. There are many bras specifically for mastectomies, both single and double. Think about the size you will be after surgery. Consider if you are going right to reconstruction, if you will have expanders, or decide to remain flat.

I would have at least two to three to switch out every few days. Personally I went with neutral colors—one nude, one black, one white—to go with anything, especially as I started to venture out and about, getting out of my pjs and into normal clothes again. SheFIT and Athleta were two brands I personally used (not affiliated), but I am sure there are a lot of great options.

2. As far as your clothes are concerned, you will want to wear comfortable, not too-tight-fitting clothes. Most likely you will not leave the house for the first few days (unless heading to the doctor) so comfy clothes or jammies are key. Also, stock up on button-up shirts and/or jammies, wide-neck shirts, and easy-to-step-into

dresses if and when you are ready to dress up a little. Once again, nothing overhead because you will not be able to raise your hands over your head for some time. For your pants or shorts, opt for elastic or drawstring. Pulling up tight pants or jeans would probably not be fun either. You are looking for comfort and items that easy to put on by yourself.

3.   Consider buying a mastectomy robe or shirts for the time that you have the drains in. These garments have drain pockets inside to hold the drains, so they are not just hanging down, which I imagine would be super uncomfortable. Also, there are drain clips you can buy separately to hold the drain tubes in place to attach to normal tops or shirts.

4.   Slip-on shoes, flip flops, or slippers will be convenient. You will not want to bend down and put on shoes, so any kind of slip-on will be helpful.

> I have created For the Love of Jugs Surgery Checklist to assist you. Go to www.fortheloveofjugs.com or access your Breastie's Meditation Guide now.

Take a Moment to Honor Your Body

Now that decisions have been made and most of the prep work is done, let's talk about honoring your body as it is right now before the changes of surgery take place.

It's inevitable your body will change with surgery, right? RIGHT.

So it is really important to take some time to honor your body before surgery. How can you do this?

There are a few ways that come to mind, but ultimately it is up to you to figure out what the best way to honor your body will be. Creating moments of sacred space allows you to pour love into your body and create a deeper appreciation for your temple. This really should be done not only before but during and after the surgery as well.

FYI: Don't forget we will discuss body image, forgiveness, and reconnecting with your body after breast cancer and surgery even more in Chapter 8. There you will find more practices to help create a beautiful bond with your body once again. For now, let's focus on appreciating and honoring your body before it changes.

For me, one of the most powerful ways to honor your body (and this may sound weird) is to take a picture of your breasts before you go into surgery. You can simply do a quick selfie or maybe even do a professional photo shoot before and after to celebrate.

I did a quick, last-minute selfie, and I am so glad I did. It took me a while to want to look at the picture, but there are now times I go back and have a moment with my body as it was before. In those moments, I create presence and send love to myself for all that I am, which signals a sense of appreciation and acceptance to my body. It immediately shifts me into a state of loving compassion and reminds me of all that I have overcome since being diagnosed.

Every time I look at that picture it reminds me of what I can do—my power, my willingness, and my commitment to myself. It is truly a sacred moment with myself.

Of course I have created another meditation for you to accompany this topic. This may be a more subtle way to honor the body but still super powerful for your energy and emotional state of being. It can be a soothing way to move from fear to love and compassion for your vessel that you live in.

> Time to access your Breastie's Meditation Guide for a beautiful visualization and meditation I created for you, the Chapter 5 meditation.

I hope this chapter gives you some sense of peace as you prepare for surgery. There is so much information out there, which may make you feel scattered and overwhelmed, both mentally and physically. My intention in this chapter is to cover all the bases in a fun and meaningful way, giving you real information from someone who has walked the walk.

Simply use this information for what it's worth, just information. Don't rush to make any decisions and make sure you are fully aligned in your next steps. As with everything we talk about in this book, it boils down to what's right for you—see what products, preparation, and information feels aligned to you and leave the rest.

Sending you love and light as you embark on your journey to recovery.

AFFIRMATION:
I OPEN MY MIND TO CHANGE
AND RELEASE CONTROL.

Breastie's Notes, Thoughts, and Ahas

How can I release the need for control and trust the process ahead?

What affirmations or practices help me embrace change with an open heart?

Chapter Six

Post Surgery

AFFIRMATION:
I AM AT PEACE WITH WHAT IS, AND I GIFT MYSELF
THE TIME TO HEAL.

Welcome home! Let's now chat about post-surgery life. I hope surgery went as well as can be expected, and you are now at home healing. Remember to give yourself the grace, love, compassion, and the time you deserve to heal. Your body has been through a lot physically, so the best thing you can do is rest and let the power of your body do its thing to heal.

The first recommendation I will offer is to not rush your healing. That reminds me of the Trevor Hall song, "You Can't Rush Your Healing." If you haven't heard that song, do yourself a favor and have a listen.

We know this is not always the easiest for most people, let alone for Type A, a.k.a. overly active people. We all can get impatient, antsy, and simply want to get back to doing things we love. Rushing our bodies and doing things too quickly can only prolong your healing and possibly add more pain and discomfort. This can even further add injury to your body. Does that sound worth it? No, I didn't think so.

I will emphasize once again I am no doctor, and most of this information is from experience—either from myself or other Pink Sisters. I am sure you will receive a list of side effects, but if you experience any fever, build up of blood, or infection at the incision or drain site, hardness, or any changes to your breasts, please immediately call your doctor's office.

Surgical Drains After a Mastectomy

Let's start with drains, drains, drains. You may have dreaded them, feared them, or you ignored them leading up to this moment, but now they are here. You may wake up from surgery with one or two on each breast depending on your surgery.

Now, if you don't already know, the main purpose of the drains is to allow any excess fluid that may build up after removing the breast to drain. They are required for most, if not all, in this type of surgery, but the downside is they may also leave the potential for bacteria to enter, which can lead to bigger issues. No matter how many you have, it is of the utmost importance to keep your drains clean and dry so you can get them removed as soon as possible without any additional issues that prolong the removal. While there is no denying their presence, the good thing is they are temporary, so why not make it a short-and-sweet relationship?

With that said, the nurses at the hospital should show you (and/or the person picking you up from the hospital) how to not only clean the drains but also how to drain the fluid. The fluid will need to drain a few times a day every day while you have them. You also will need to keep track of how much fluid you dump into the measuring cup from each drain, every time you dump them.

I have created a special drain tracker for you that is included your Breastie's Meditation Guide. Hopefully you have downloaded by now, but if not head over to www.fortheloveofjugs.com.

Please for the love, do not slack in keeping up with this list of information because your doctors will ask. This allows them to better understand how the fluid is draining and when they can remove the drains.

Just a note: The fluid will start to get less and less, and the color may start to change as the days go by. That's normal but again something to track. And if you are wondering, removing the drains does not really hurt; for me it was painless and quick. Hopefully that is the same experience for you.

I know you will be very happy once they are removed but, in the meantime, try not to create too much negative energy around the inconvenience while you have them. We know how a negative mindset can bring you down, right? Instead, shift to a higher vibe and be thankful for them as they remove excess fluid and help you heal. Like I said, there is no denying their presence, but it is only temporary.

Affirm that with me: This is all temporary. Repeat it over and over until you feel the shift.

Pain

I am not gonna lie. In most cases, I do not usually take medication, but I did take the pain medication they provided me for at least the first few days after my surgeries. You may be totally different and not experience pain the way I did. See how your body reacts, but don't try to be a hero and push through any pain.

I am not here to tell you what to do or not to do, but I say do whatever you need to be as comfortable as possible. If you choose to take pain medication following your surgery, keep a pen and paper by your bedside to track the time so you don't wait too long, reducing any onset of pain. I would also keep pretzels, crackers, or a granola bar on hand when you take the medication to reduce any nausea. And don't forget to keep up with your fiber and hydration as well to reduce any constipation and keep things smooth flowing, literally!

Lymphedema

I could probably have written a whole book about this section, but I will try to keep it short and sweet, to the point, and easy to understand. Not only do I want to help you if you experience lymphedema during your journey, but I also want to inform you of the importance of the lymphatic system since your lymphatic system can be compromised after breast surgery and/or radiation if lymph nodes have been removed. I want to be clear, I am not specialized in lymphatic drainage massage techniques, but I have become quite the lymph nerd and know a great deal about the lymphatic system.

Let's first start with an overview of the lymphatic system and how important it is to your health before we dive into lymphedema. This information is important for everyone to know and understand—whether you have experienced a cancer diagnosis or not.

What is the lymph system?

The lymph system is our body's detoxification network, which is closely tied to the immune system and the cardiovascular system. Basically, it moves lymph fluid, the clear fluid of the lymphatic system that not only carries immune boosting fighter cells, but also excess waste such as cancer cells, proteins, and hormones. The fluid moves through specific channels like your lymph nodes (which are most commonly known), but also capillaries, trunks, and ducts that are all throughout the body. The fluid eventually makes its way back to the heart and through the bloodstream to be eliminated.

Interestingly enough, unlike the cardiovascular system, which has the heart to pump blood through, the lymphatic system has no pump. You are the pump, which to me is super cool and empowering. So when you exercise, get massages, swim, or jump, you are encouraging lymphatic drainage. Seems pretty easy breezy.

However, like I mentioned above, your lymphatic system can be compromised during a cancer diagnosis or after something major like surgery, radiation, and removal of the lymph nodes. Since removing lymph nodes disrupts our lymphatic pathway to detoxification, it becomes a perfect storm for lymphedema to occur.

What is lymphedema exactly?

I am glad you asked, because before breast cancer I didn't really know. Well, to be honest, I didn't know truly how powerful and important the whole lymphatic system was until I started learning more about it. Now I have turned into a lymph fanatic.

Basically, lymphedema is your body's signal that the lymph fluid is not draining properly, leading to swelling (or a back up) in the body. With breast cancer specifically, the axillary lymph nodes region (just under the arm) is the common area for node removal because this area drains the breast, arm, chest and neck. Lymphedema is most likely to occur with the more nodes you have removed due to bacterial infection, lack of movement, radiation scarring, or surgery. These are just a few of the culprits that can increase the risk of lymphedema. Keep in mind this can happen right away, after surgery/radiation, or even possibly up to three years after. Thankfully in most situations, lymphedema is a temporary condition but serious nonetheless.

What should you look out for?

Some symptoms of lymphedema are swelling in your arm or hand, feeling of tightness or pain, bras not fitting like they did recently, or a weakness in the arm. Please be sure to let your doctor know if you experience any of these right away, because there are ways to reduce some symptoms and many specialists to guide you, especially during treatment. No need to suffer, especially when most treatments for lymphedema and/or any preventative treatments are natural and you just need the right specialist to help.

Prevention is key when it comes to the lymphatic system and reducing the risk of lymphedema. There are many things I love about the lymphatic system, but what's really cool is that you can incorporate some natural (and free) ways to assist it. Obviously double check with your team of doctors first, and if okay with your doctor, I recommend starting these sooner than later. And maybe encourage some of your loved ones to join you!

1. Move your body. Here we are again talking about exercise! Exercises like swimming, walking, strength training or jumping can help move the lymph fluid. As I mentioned before in this book, moving our body is important and now helping the lymphatic system is another huge benefit. Moving encourages the fluid to move towards the lymphatic pathways leading back towards the heart and eventually detoxifying excess hormones, cancer cells, and proteins. Clearly right after surgery you may not be able to incorporate exercises right away, but do what you can. Even simply walking is a great way to get things moving in the body.

2. Lymphatic massage. Manual Lymphatic Drainage (MLD) massage is a special technique that requires a licensed certification. Do not go to any massage therapist; find a specialized MLD technician in your area. Maybe even better, check your local area for a massage therapist who specializes in breast health and lymphedema for Pink Sisters.
3. Breath-work. Diaphragmatic breath-work also helps move the lymph fluid deep in the body and gut, whereas movement or massage might not be able to access them.
4. Compression garments. Wearing compression sleeves may also reduce risk of lymphedema swelling. It helps apply pressure to move the fluid rather than it staying stagnant.
5. Reduce inflammation through hydration and diet.

Story Time

I remember a few weeks after my reconstruction surgery, I was getting ready to go down to the Florida Keys for a quick trip with some of my girlfriends, and I noticed some discomfort the night before in my left breast.

When I woke up the next morning to shower, my left breast was super tender and much bigger than my right. I knew something was not right! In somewhat of a panic, I called my doctor's office to explain what I was experiencing and get their opinion. They, of course, wanted to see me right away. While I was relieved they wanted to see me, my emotions went right to frustration and sadness because all I wanted to do was go away with my girls and not think about cancer for a few days!

I thought, *Thanks, cancer, you are holding me back again and now I won't be able to go!* Tears streamed down my cheeks as I called my friends to tell them to go without me. I was in disbelief this was happening.

I saw my plastic surgeon first, and he said I would need to see my breast surgeon who, thankfully, was just down the hall. As soon as I walked out of the plastic surgeon's office, I saw my breast surgeon heading into the office with his scrubs on as if he was going into surgery. He saw me walking towards him, and I immediately grabbed his attention to tell him my situation.

It was divine timing to say the least because he mentioned he was supposed to be in surgery, but the patient was running late and it just so happened he ran up to the office for a few minutes. After seeing the panic in my face, he ushered me right into the ultrasound room to find it was thankfully just a seroma and nothing too serious.

Seromas are common after surgery and basically fluid build up near the incision site. Usually they can be left untreated because the body just reabsorbs the fluid, but he was able to drain it due to how much discomfort I was in. He sent me on my way, and I was able to make it to the girls trip and had a wonderful time.

I tell you this story to give you just one more reminder to listen to your body and do what you need to when something doesn't feel right. This may come up, and I hope hearing my story can reduce a freak-out moment like I had.

* * *

As you can see, there are many ways to reduce lymphedema or any other complications. However, as you saw with the seroma I experienced, there are no safeguards to fully prevent them. The only thing you can do is to incorporate the preventative suggestions into your daily routine and do your best. Things will pop up so you have to be ready.

In true *For the Love of Jugs* mentality, I want you to be extra in-tune with your body and on heightened alert to notice any excess swelling, especially in the breast or arm where the lymph nodes were removed. It is essential to contact your doctor or a specialist if you do, so they can help you right away to reduce further complications.

Caring for Your Incisions and Scar Care

Now on to your incisions and scar care. Clearly what type of surgery you experienced will determine where and how many scars you may have. Once your drains are removed, there are no more worries of getting them wet, and you can enjoy showering and have freedom once again. Yay!

However, try to keep the heat down by showering with warm water instead of scalding hot water. Then simply pat dry the incision site rather than rubbing the area dry. This may all sound redundant and obvious, but keeping the incision site clean is super important for reducing infections.

They will look worse before they look better; they may be darker than normal or red with potential bruising especially in the beginning. While most likely your scars are in an area that will be covered ninety percent of the time, it is super important that you care for them properly to make sure they heal as best as they can.

What should you do for your healing and scar care?

○ First, there are many creams and ointments that help, but wait until the stitches are out. I loved using vitamin E and castor oil since both are natural products and easy to find. I am sure there are special creams curated specifically for scars if a more specialized product is your jam. If you choose to go that route, remember to look for clean products without chemicals and toxic ingredients.

○ Silicone sheets, which you can buy from most drug stores, may help the coloring and appearance of your scars.

○ Massage your scars once you get approval from your doctor. Massaging the scars can help reduce inflammation, reduce pain, and help repair the fascia in the area.

○ Reduce inflammatory foods, alcohol, and high amounts of sodium. Take in foods rich in vitamins A, C, E, and zinc such as spinach, oranges, bell peppers, mushrooms, and legumes.

Today, I look at my scars as a reminder of my strength and all I have endured, but that didn't happen overnight. It has taken me years to be proud of my scars. And still to this day, I make sure my bathing suits, shirts, and sports bras do not show my scars, especially the one where the cancer was.

While it makes me proud, I clearly still have some healing to do before showing them to the world. I only say this because I want you to understand your healing is not immediate. It will take time and effort to heal yourself on all levels surrounding different areas of your journey. As I mentioned, we will talk more about body image and accepting your body in Chapter 8 where I will give you some practices to help you love your body again, scars, and new boobies too! Stay tuned.

For now, as we finish up this chapter on surgery, we see life may not be so glamorous at the moment. Between drains, scars, and possibly nippleless breasts, there is a lot to overcome and you already have endured so much up until this point. However, like all things, this too shall pass and you are one day closer to full recovery and hopefully becoming cancer free.

Take one day at a time, put one foot in front of the other, and remember not rush your healing!

"Never be ashamed of a scar. It only means you are stronger than whatever tried to hurt you." -Unknown

AFFIRMATION:
I AM AT PEACE WITH WHAT IS, AND I GIFT MYSELF
THE TIME TO HEAL.

Breastie's Notes, Thoughts, and Ahas

What does giving myself the gift of time and peace to heal mean to me?

How can I honor my recovery process with patience and compassion?

Chapter Seven

Radiation

AFFIRMATION:
I CAN DO HARD THINGS THROUGH A LOVING AND
COMPASSIONATE CONNECTION WITH MY BODY.

The chronological time frame where radiation falls in your journey (if at all) may differ just like chemo and surgery paths. I personally did not experience radiation, so instead of acting like I know what I am talking about, I called on my Pink Sisters to help me with this chapter.

With that said, this chapter may have a different vibe than other chapters because it is their stories, in their words. If radiation is part of your journey, please continue reading. Their stories are real, authentic, completely vulnerable, and I am truly grateful for their help in this project.

Jan's Experience

Jan had twenty-eight days of radiation and, for her, the radiation part went really quick, because it only takes about ten minutes and it's every day, so it goes quickly. She had some sunburn and sensitivity on her skin, but never to the point of it breaking the skin or dealing with open wounds.

Her doctors did mention to keep specific ointments on the radiated area to help condition the skin. Her skin did change color where the radiation was done.

She also said that the after-effects felt worse than when actually going through it; at least they were for her. She found that her breast was distorted because of the radiation. She noticed that there are certain movements, like reaching for something, and she gets a sharp pain where the radiation was. There are times when she wonders what the long-term effects will be.

Jan also noticed that between the chemo and possibly the radiation, she feels more joint issues than she has in her whole life. Her flexibility and joints have deteriorated, and that seems to be the hardest part because she has always been active, always pushing herself, and now she feels limited. Unfortunately, working out or being active simply hurts.

For Jan, it's hard to tell what affected her more because the radiation started within thirty days from chemo ending. Was it the chemo or the radiation? We may never know.

I asked if she had to pick between the two, which would she pick?

Jan said, "Radiation seemed like a breeze compared to going through the chemo."

Tina's Experience

Tina was recommended to add radiation to her journey after chemotherapy and two lumpectomy surgeries. As I think most women are, Tina was a bit scared and intimidated by radiation, but she felt it was something she really needed to do.

At the time, she did feel some emotional distress but not sure if it was due to the uncertainty of a new treatment or underlying effects of the chemo she just finished.

Her body was definitely tired physically and emotionally. Thankfully the physician and his staff were so kind, gentle, and supportive that it made it doable.

I asked her if there were any recommendations regarding supplements, diet, or creams to add during the process. A doctor may recommend a specific cream to use multiple times a day to reduce redness, burning, and distorting of the radiated area.

Tina did not experience too many limitations other than not submerging under water if there are any blisters or open wounds. She did experience some redness during radiation, but that is now minimal.

Interestingly enough, she lost the majority of her hair during chemo, but once she started radiation, whatever hair on her body she still had completely came out. Tina does still have some range-of-motion limitations to this day, which could either be from scar tissue from her lumpectomies or the radiation. Again, not sure which is the culprit.

Other than that, she does not seem to have any long-term effects, as of right now.

Tina also mentioned she would do it again, so I asked her what advice she would give to other Pink Sisters. She says to just trust the process. Trust the radiologist, use the creams suggested, and hydrate, hydrate, hydrate (so important)!

One of the most healing moments she experienced, after about a week after completing radiation, was going to the ocean and taking a dip to let the saltwater help to heal internally and externally. If you cannot make it to the ocean, then take a salt bath. Add a cupful of table salt into a warm bath and soak as long as you can. (Please do not do this if you have open wounds or blisters).

Brynn's Experience

When she was prescribed thirty-three radiation treatments after chemotherapy, she didn't expect it to be one of the hardest parts of her journey. She shares that she would rather go through chemo again than face radiation. It was supposed to be quick, a ten-minute treatment, in and out. But for Brynn, it rarely went that smoothly. Instead, she found herself spending hours at the clinic, waiting, frustrated, often in tears, and yes, angry.

She mentioned, "That radiation also has a cumulative effect no one warns you about. At first, you feel like you can handle it. But slowly, over time, it wears you down. Out of nowhere, you're hit with this overwhelming fatigue—you have zero energy left. The exhaustion creeps up on you, and before you know it, getting out of bed feels like an Olympic feat."

That's when she learned that rest wasn't just helpful—it was necessary.

As a twenty-seven-year-old working to keep her health insurance, Brynn was constantly trying to balance work and treatment. More often than not, she was the youngest person in the room and seemingly the only one who was in a hurry to get in and out. There were days when she questioned whether she could keep going back. But she did. And each day, she had to stand up for herself to make sure she wasn't sitting there for hours.

For anyone facing radiation, she wants you to know, "It's okay to feel frustrated; it's okay to cry; and it's okay to be angry. But don't give up. Most importantly, rest. Even when it feels unbearable, trust that you're moving forward with one treatment at a time."

* * *

First off, I want to thank my three beautiful and vulnerable friends who have shared their stories! I know how difficult it is to go back in time and bring up old memories that we sometimes would like to forget.

In all three stories, I noticed a theme with radiation, much similar to chemo. There seems to be a pattern with a sense of nervousness about the unknown; side effects are no fun; the power of listening to your body; and hydration and rest are back in the hot seat for their utmost importance!

Similar to my chemo experience, wouldn't you agree?

With all of that said, my intention is to show you that everyone's experiences are different and two are never the exact same. Like many Pink Sisters who came before you, you will have your own personal story to write. No matter if you go through radiation, chemo, or surgery—it seems the treatment does not matter, it's the way you approach your journey.

Go into it with an open mind, prepare your body, and stand in your power!

You can do hard things, but in true *For the Love of Jugs* manner, do it with ease in your MBHS.

You got this, Pink Sister!

AFFIRMATION:
I CAN DO HARD THINGS THROUGH A LOVING AND COMPASSIONATE CONNECTION WITH MY BODY.

Breastie's Notes, Thoughts, and Ahas

How can I maintain a loving and compassionate relationship with my body during hard times?

What are small ways I can show gratitude to my body for its strength?

Chapter Eight

Your Body Is a Temple

AFFIRMATION:
I AM PERFECTLY IMPERFECT, AND I AM BEAUTIFUL
INSIDE AND OUT.

Even though I wrote a lot about acceptance way back in the first chapter, it was mainly with regards to accepting the diagnosis and your mental state. The topic of acceptance is so important that I feel we should discuss it again because of the many different layers of acceptance.

Let's talk about body acceptance. I bet from time to time, even before your diagnosis, you would shame yourself for looking a certain way. Am I right?

Accept Your Changing Body

I feel this is one of the most important chapters in this book. I mean they all are in their own way, but this one in particular because, regardless of a cancer diagnosis or not, we are typically harder on ourselves than anyone else. Women especially.

First it's important to go backward before we can go forward in acceptance and creating a strong, loving bond with your body again. I know loving your body can seem hard to embrace after a breast cancer diagnosis because it may feel like your body let you down.

Your body did not let you down.

There are many factors within your cancer diagnosis that have helped weaken your body for cancer to congregate and form. Stop thinking your body let you down!

There are other things out of our control that do let us down. From the greed within the pharmaceutical companies, food industry, and medical world, to the environmental toxins and constant overload of electronic devices—all of which do not help our bodies to stop cancer from expressing. I do not want to go on another rampage about this, but I mention it because it is not your fault!

I need you to understand that your body did not let you down, so change the narrative in your mind to guide you back toward a loving connection and better relationship with your body. In doing so, we know it helps the healing process on all levels.

Let's release the negative vibes, see past the imperfections, and learn what it feels like to truly love our bodies. Sound like a plan?

Body image is usually a pain point that may feel super triggering for any woman, at any age, let alone someone going through a cancer diagnosis. The body gets such a hard rap during all of this because it is the first line of attack.

Let's face it. There is this underlying idea of having to be perfect, look perfect or flawless, and it is undeniably everywhere. Especially with smartphones attached to almost every human! The constant information at our fingertips shows us images of women trying to lose weight for the perfect body. Or anti-aging products everywhere because we are afraid of wrinkles and aging naturally, etc.

In general, women feel this pressure, but now add cancer treatments that make our skin look gray or drab, give us burns on our breasts, make us bald, make us lose too much weight, or make us gain weight, etc. There is no doubt body dysmorphia is a real thing and may be exacerbated after cancer treatments.

> I want you to think about this: It's not the body thinking you are too heavy, or the scars are ugly, or your breasts are not even. No, it's the mind choosing to harp on the idea of the imperfections making you less than and not the imperfections themselves.

Read that again.

Our minds harp on the idea of imperfections and not the imperfections themselves. Our brain is the thinker and the meaning-maker that makes meaning out of the imperfections and then labels all the imperfections as bad.

The body feels all of these negative thoughts and vibes that our minds create (again not our bodies), which is what leads us to anxiety, low self esteem, depression, and added stress.

By the way, aren't these the exact things that we want to get rid of on our road to recovery? So why are we so fixated on being perfect? Stop trying to be perfect!

There is not one thing in this world that is perfect, so why pressure our bodies to look perfect or be perfect?

Your body went through so much; it is time to show it the love it deserves. Let's dive deeper into how we can love our bodies again and quiet the mind's expectations.

> What if I said, "Your body is a temple."
>   How does that make you feel when you read that sentence?

Do you appreciate your body and see your body as a temple after the diagnosis, or are you completely disconnected from your body?

I am sure it's the latter.

Basically, the desire to have a perfect, healthy body, in turn, blocks us from fully loving who we are and what we look like in the present moment.

A dear friend of mine once said, "You cannot heal a body that you hate."

Whoa, that hit me hard.

The definition of hate is intense or passionate dislike. Ultimately to hate is truly a form of disapproval and not accepting what is. I believe hate is a super strong word and one I do not typically have in my vocabulary.

If we constantly tear ourselves down, then that unfortunately is a form of hate in my eyes.

How can we hate our bodies? How can we hate anything about ourselves?

We are beautiful beings who were given this one vessel to go through life. We are one in a trillion!

Yet we shame, sabotage, and sometimes disconnect from not only our bodies but the essence of who we are. Not to mention, shaming our bodies for years and years only enhances any imbalances in our overall holistic well-being, which ultimately leads to sickness in the physical body.

> Instead of shaming our body, how can we love and respect our bodies so we create a healthy inner environment to thrive after cancer? It's called self-compassion and self-worth!

And when you couple self-worth with compassion, wow, it can create a game-changing vibe in your life. I want you to understand that you are worthy of loving yourself, your whole self, including your body and the changes that occur. I want you to see your body as the strong, beautiful temple it is.

It's time to set aside the idea of being perfect and appreciate all that you are right here, right now! You are alive. Isn't that something worth celebrating?

Instead of wasting time harping on all your imperfections, pause to appreciate all that you are—Mind, Body, Heart, and Soul.

Remember you cannot heal what you hate, so it's time to shift your mindset and start appreciating your imperfections, seeing your body through a compassionate lens.

Do you recall how in the beginning of this book, we decided to shift our mindset from scarcity, fear, and negative vibes toward positivity, love, and compassion? Well, this theme needs to continue through reconnecting back to your body.

Now that we are this far into the book, can we agree that you know that remaining in a negative head space about the way you look, the changes you endured, and/or comparing yourself to how you used to look is not a good place to be in?

I hope I have instilled this concept lovingly into your mind by now, but just in case there is still doubt, here is another reminder.

> Release the negative vibes of having to be perfect or exactly like you were before, and see your body through a lens of love to shift towards appreciation. Valuing not only who you were before but, more importantly, who you are now.

We all constantly change physically, energetically, and emotionally from moment to moment, day to day, procedure to procedure.

Who I am today is different from who I was yesterday.

You are different than you were yesterday.

Our thoughts, our cells, our emotions change too, so allow yourself to take a moment to honor who you are and what you look like right now with love and compassion.

* * *

These next few practices can be extremely powerful and the catalyst to help you shift your views on your body after breast cancer. They will encourage you to be vulnerable and honest with yourself.

First we will acknowledge what your triggers are, then shift how you see yourself and the thoughts you think. This will help you to embody the MBHS connection to move toward a loving relationship with your body.

It's important to understand that what you see in the mirror prompts what you think and say about your body, which all need to be in sync towards a positive, affirming, aligned place.

Now let's approach the next few practices with an open mind and a clear heart.

Acknowledge Your Triggers

We all know that acceptance can significantly shift our perception of ourselves, but in order to see yourself differently you kinda need to know what your triggers are.

What makes you feel self conscious? What makes you not fill yourself up with the love and the compassion you deserve?

It's essential to identify and acknowledge your trigger spots so we know what needs to shift. Is it the scars, the implants, the missing nipples, the radiation burns, the missing hair, the feeling your body let you down? Is it something even prior to treatment that had you feeling less than beautiful? Why do you not see your body as anything other than beautiful and powerful?

This practice may feel a bit heavy at first, but it is just about acknowledging what specifically sends you into a spiral of negative thoughts or actions towards your body. I want you to see this simply as a practice of observation or self inquiry rather than attaching any meaning to what comes up.

Now it may be simple in theory but not necessarily an easy practice, so be gentle with yourself during this process.

We are going to do a writing exercise in a moment, but this might be a good time to regulate yourself first.

First, open your Breastie's Meditation Guide to listen to the Chapter 8 meditation before the next steps.

Now, time to grab a pen and flip to the blank pages at the end of this chapter.

I want you to ask yourself, *What do I not like about my body?*

Try not to let that question make you go completely numb or blocked. Allow all answers to come up—all of them.

It's also completely normal if this brings up an array of jumbled answers and a busy mind. This is the perfect time to get real honest and vulnerable with yourself. I want you to know that you are safe to "go there" in your mind.

Repeat after me: I am safe to witness my triggers and acknowledge what blocks me from loving my whole self.

You are safe to bring forth all of the nonsense in your mind about your body. Let your mind go and think about everything you do not like about yourself, but here's the kicker: Whatever you do, please do not judge yourself in the process. Easier said than done, I know, but try not to judge yourself!

- ◦ Start writing down everything that comes up. It does not need to make sense, just throw it on the paper. As you write, start to notice how the mind wants to take over your thoughts with either giving negative meaning, labeling, shaming, or name calling, etc.
- ◦ Recognize this as just your ego stepping in to tell you that you are not good enough.
- ◦ Remind yourself that is not the truth. Your self-worth, love, and compassion need to interject and remind you of your beauty.
- ◦ Remember the affirmation for this chapter: I am perfectly imperfect, and I am beautiful inside and out. Repeat this over and over to shift your thoughts.

You deserve your own love and are an absolute beautiful being who needs to reconnect and find your way back to loving yourself and your body. We need to create new patterns to learn to accept, love, nourish, and constantly not only cherish our changing bodies but accept all we went through during life. That takes daily effort. In the beginning it will feel uncomfortable, which is expected, just know that this work takes time.

I want to be fully transparent. It took me a hot minute to accept the differences in my body and welcome my new boobies. Like months, maybe even years.

And yet, sometimes, I still have moments of disassociation and think negative thoughts about my body and breasts. Thankfully, with the work around acceptance and gratitude, those moments are few and far between; however, they do pop in now and then.

For instance, one night I found myself harping on the rippling of the implants. The difference now is, after the inner work, I do not stay in that negative zone for too long. I consciously pull myself out of the negative head-space and shift my views, thoughts, and actions thus bringing me back to a place of compassion and appreciation.

Mirror Work and Releasing Judgment

After you acknowledge what triggers you, then you can move on to this next practice: mirror work. I gotta say this one was probably the most powerful and vulnerable practices that helped me towards accepting my new breasts.

> Remember you cannot heal what you hate. I am actually adding to that statement: You cannot heal what you cannot accept.

Let me explain.

Shortly after my surgery, I covered up and did not want to look at my breasts. I was definitely not accepting my new breasts. I knew I needed to shift my views and mindset of how I viewed my body. To help my acceptance, I stood in front of the mirror in my bathroom or closet, before or after a shower, naked, and just stared at my body and breasts. Uncomfortable at first to say the least! Sometimes I cried; sometimes I laughed; and sometimes I felt stuck—numb to the core in disbelief that this was my life.

However, in time, it got easier. I felt more comfortable staring at my body. I learned to appreciate myself as I was in that moment. All of those moments allowed raw emotions to come through and create beautiful, honest, vulnerable experiences with myself. I know it sounds weird, but the mirror work encouraged some serious healing, which even continues today!

Give it a try. Maybe even do this before your surgery as well.

1. Stand in front of the mirror naked.
2. Take the time to really observe your breasts. Observing without judgment simply noticing the size, firmness, scars, dimples and indentations, your nipples or the place where your nipples were, etc. Don't think your way through this; just observe with your eyes and let the emotions roll as they come up.
3. Don't hold back. Cry if you need to; scream if you need to; laugh if you need to. Just feel through this practice and accept all that is in this present moment without attachment or judgment.

4. Stay there as long as you need. Don't rush it.
5. If you feel called to write more in this book or a jour-
    nal, write down what you feel to help fully release the
    feels from your body and energy.

This work can be powerful and cathartic in your healing.
Remember you can't fully heal what you hate or what you
cannot accept, so if you are not connecting to your new
breasts and body, then you are suppressing. Whatever emotions you are suppressing will express at some point, like a
ticking time bomb, so release, release, release.

Keep in mind this work is not a one-and-done, and voila!
you love everything you see. You might find you need to do
this mirror work multiple times before your mind shifts what
it sees. There is no magic number.

Try this anytime you feel less than about your body because let's be honest, your body is changing and your emotions come and go, so it is your duty to shift from judgment
to love and acceptance for your changing body. You deserve
it!

Internal Dialogue and Body Image

Okay, let's move on to creating awareness around your in-
ternal dialogue and how you speak to yourself.

I read this amazing quote from an unknown author, "Every
cell in your body is eavesdropping on your thoughts."

From what I've learned from yoga and various books and
podcasts, our bodies are always listening. Negative or toxic
thoughts can weigh heavy on us, which ultimately leads towards stress and trauma, leaving an imprint in our bodies.

And not a good one. The way you talk to yourself is yet another important piece of the puzzle towards acceptance and healing. Can you agree that you cannot move towards love and compassion about your body if your mind is constantly repeating, *I hate the way my boobs are or why am I so fat?*

Let's look at it from another angle.

Would you ever say half the things you think about your body to your best friend or child? I bet that is a big fat no. Change the narrative and imagine having a more empowering, inspiring, positive self-talk like you would with your best friend, shall we?

Awareness is the first step to any type of change. The goal is to be aware as the negative Nelly thoughts appear. If you become aware of those thoughts before or during the process, then you are conscious enough to change the thought and shift to a positive, loving thought.

I want you to really connect to your thoughts and notice when the conversation in your head, especially about yourself, starts to get negative or judgey, and take note of how it feels in your body.

* * *

Girl, you know I love me some affirmations. As you have already experienced, affirmations can serve as a great disruptor and change from a negative to a positive tone, not only in the mind, but in the body too. This also starts to rewire some of your neurons and change the way the brain reacts, making positive thoughts more common.

Below are a few affirmations/statements that may help you. If none call out to you, then you go back to the core value affirmations you created in Chapter 1.

Fun fact: Writing them on your mirror is a fun way to incorporate this shift, and you can add this to the mirror work practice as well. Either way, using one or two affirmations to interrupt the negative vibes in the moment creates a loving, positive environment in your mind and body for a big impact.

If you are a bit overwhelmed or stressed before this practice, then pause to regulate. I want to make sure you come from a regulated place. As you know, if you are stressed and negative, just saying a few positive sentences in your mind may not feel as powerful. And I know you want to get as much of an impact as possible, right?

Affirmations:

I accept my body and embrace all of its beauty and its flaws.

I embody the beautiful being that I am.

I radiate from the inside out.

I send love and compassion to all parts of me.

I am beautiful, and I shine so bright for the universe to see.

I am perfectly imperfect.

I am one sexy being.

* * *

I'm curious: Did this chapter make you feel a little uncomfortable or empowered?

My hope is this chapter has empowered you to change your relationship with how you view your body but also encouraged you to experience some (or many) of uncomfortable moments too.

Let's start to sum things up.

The highlights of this chapter are acknowledgment, acceptance, and embodiment. Acknowledge your triggers, accept yourself, and embody the love, respect, and dedication your body deserves.

Truth is we cannot be different, think different, or act different if we stay the same. Change happens at the speed of uncomfortability, so in order to step out of your comfort zone, you have to allow for some uncomfortable moments to create new norms.

Truth is it's uncomfortable to stare at ourselves, be our own cheerleader, and be honest with ourselves, but it shouldn't be. It's totally okay to feel uncomfortable, and I hope you feel more empowered as you do this work. I would love to see that as our new normal!

I promise you the more you do these practices, the easier it gets. These practices really helped me re-establish a beautiful bond with my body. Now, I would be lying if I said those negative thoughts don't creep in every so often, but when I find myself doubting my body or feeling down about it, I reach into my little box of practices that I shared above and hit the reset button. Afterwards, I feel more appreciative and grateful, which allows me to see my body as the beautiful temple that it is, scars and all!

I want you to see yourself as the beautiful, strong queen that you are. You are beautiful inside and out. You radiate beauty even though you may not feel it during your journey.

It is within you because You are You! You are a miracle and worthy of seeing your own beauty. You have been through so much, and now it is important to tap into love, appreciation, and compassion with regards to who you are in this moment. Allow yourself to release the attachments and labels of perfection, so you can view your temple as the radiant vessel you were lucky enough to inhabit. This is where true healing can happen.

If you feel you need additional support with body image or any of the topics we have discussed in this book, I encourage you to seek professional help. A cancer diagnosis can feel heavy and traumatic, and while all of this information is amazing, sometimes we do need outside help to guide us through our healing. If that speaks to you, then I encourage you to find someone who believes in holistic healing to help you through this Mind, Body, Heart, and Soul (MBHS) process.

AFFIRMATION:
I AM PERFECTLY IMPERFECT, AND I AM BEAUTIFUL INSIDE AND OUT.

Breastie's Notes, Thoughts, and Ahas

How do I define beauty for myself beyond physical appearance?

What are three things I appreciate about my body today?

Chapter Nine

THRIVE Don't Just Survive

**"THE WOUND IS THE PLACE
WHERE THE LIGHT ENTERS YOU." - RUMI**

Okay, Breastie, we are now at the end of the book. My hope is that you have not only picked up a great deal of helpful information for your cancer journey but have created some amazing new habits and found a whole new love and appreciation for yourself during our time together.

All of the spiritual practices, information, affirmations, journaling prompts, and a whole lot of ahas! were provided to help you heal, get stronger, and more connected to self—not only for your cancer journey but in life as well. Because, at some point, the treatments, doctors appointments, and scans will subside, and I do not want you to fall back into your old ways. All along, I have nudged you to reduce the noise of fear, be present every day, and tap into your power with one goal in mind: Thrive with grace and ease.

174

This goes for wherever you are in your journey whether just diagnosed, finishing treatment, years out of treatment, or you have a lifetime of treatments. Regardless of the stage, I believe it is imperative to continue the inner work towards creating a beautiful, dynamic, harmonious, and thriving environment after cancer.

> While I pray there comes a time when your doctor clears you, hopefully pronouncing you in remission, no evidence of cancer (NED), or cancer free, I know this may not be the scenario for some of our metastatic Pink Sisters. Before I continue, let's take a moment to honor our meta Pink Baddies! Treatments may continue for a lifetime, but this is a reminder to not give in or give up! Keep going, Pink Sisters! Keep loving on your bodies, holding your heads high, feeling your feelings, and creating a peaceful environment to continue healing through your journey. I cheer for you every step of the way. Together we rise!

With that said, in true fear fashion, fear loves to surprise you when you least expect it. Remember my girl's trip/seroma story? Fear will always look for the perfect opportunity to interFEAR with your power and your peace.

You see what I did there?

Fear always loves to interrupt life and stir up some drama, but even more so when you enter back into life after treatments. This may also happen as soon as treatments start to slow down.

You might notice a slow, trickle effect of overwhelm or anxiousness coming back as you navigate life again. Very similar to the beginning of your diagnosis, the aftermath of cancer may once again drag you back into the rabbit hole of 'What ifs?' and fearful scenarios. Consuming your mind with stressful thoughts such as, *How do I ensure cancer doesn't come back?* or *How do I live a life of freedom and not one in constant fear of recurrence?* or *Where do I even start?* may have you second-guessing yourself or overthinking what you are or are not doing to reduce a cancer comeback.

Fear loves to put us in a state of lack or separation from our essence, which then gives it a louder voice than our own intuition and power. But as a *For Love of Jugs* Breastie, you know this is not the path you take, especially when you fought so hard to get where you are today.

My motto: Water where you want to grow!

If you waste your time thinking about the cancer coming back or metastasizing, then guess what? It might! It gives cancer the voice and the power—once again putting you in a low-lying frequency rather than high vibin' thrivership.

Listen, there are no guarantees on how life will play out! However, we know this fear-based mindset can be disempowering. All the more reason to stay in tune with the MBHS connection and not let fear interrupt.

Choosing to interrupt the fear and focus on building a loving and stress-free environment (both internally and externally) creates harmony in your being, and that is where we thrive. Remember, you are powerful beyond measure when your MBHS are one, so it's crucial to stay in alignment with your healing and not let fear take over.

So are you ready to thrive? At this point in our Breastie relationship, the answer better be a "Hell Yeah!"

Now that you are pumped up to thrive, let's discuss the term cancer survivor vs. thriver for a second.

We have all heard the term 'cancer survivor'. It's everywhere, right?

You may already even refer to yourself as a cancer survivor. This is a mainstream term and has been normalized because for decades, the medical world automatically sees you as a survivor the moment you are diagnosed.

Personally, I always thought one could call himself/herself a survivor after treatments finished, but nope, not the case.

The definition of survivor is a person who survives, especially a person remaining alive after an event in which others have died.

So while yes, you have technically survived cancer because your body did not succumb to cancer, and thankfully you are here today reading this amazing book. Cancer is the event in which we all survived, and quite honestly to survive just feels like a powerless, bare-minimum way of life. Do you agree?

For me, it makes me feel weak and less than powerful—like I am clutching to something outside of myself just to survive in this crazy thing called life. Don't get me wrong, there definitely may be days where you feel like all you can do is survive because of side effects or lack of energy, and that's okay. However, over time you want those days few and far between.

I am starting a new movement. Time to flip the script and call ourselves cancer thrivers. I urge you to hop on board the thriver train as well. Switch to cancer thriver and get inspired to live your best and healthiest life moving forward because you are worth it. Simply put, I believe the cancer survivor label needs to go buh BYE!

What does it take to become a thriver?

I am glad you asked. There is a huge difference between merely surviving and thriving. To thrive is a choice.

A thriver is someone who chooses to continue through life after a traumatic experience consciously and willing to make changes to their lifestyle and live a healthy life of joy and ease.

It means taking back the power in your life and living with strength, empowerment, mindfulness, wholeness, and worthiness. It means becoming your own advocate, teacher, student, and the love of your life. It means not looking outside of yourself for healing. It means opening your eyes to learning more about how you can support yourself in every aspect of your life. It means being more proactive about your overall health and well being.

It means loving yourself as a whole Mind, Body, Heart, and Soul.

Whoa, now that gives me Life!

It gives me an electrical charge running through my body. It gives me all the feels knowing I have the power within to live a life from a different point of view and perspective, especially after the impact of a cancer diagnosis. In true *For the Love of Jugs* mentality, thriving after cancer puts you back in the driver seat of your life, instead of just going through the motions waiting for the other shoe to drop.

Doesn't all of that sound amazing (well, not waiting for the shoe to drop)? Yes, the answer must be yes!

You have to drive the change you want to see. Remember in the last chapter we discussed how it takes tapping into compassion and your self-worth in order to thrive after cancer? Well, now is your time! You deserve to treat yourself like the goddess you are and THRIVE.

Thriving Lifestyle

Whether you currently have routine checkups and scans to track tumor markers or you are already out of treatment, typically you are not guided by your doctors on how to thrive after cancer. Well, unless you took my advice early on and you started to incorporate an integrative approach in your healing. Regardless, in order to thrive moving forward, changes need to be made to your lifestyle.

Why must we change after cancer?

Clearly something wasn't working before your diagnosis.

It comes down to this: It's essential to create a harmonious environment where cancer does not want to grow. Not just physically, but emotionally and energetically too, as discussed in Chapter 2. I bring this up again because, like I said, most doctors may not talk much about this topic once treatments are over. There is little-to-no guidance given on what to eat or not to eat, how to maintain a regulated nervous system, what types of supplements help your body perform the way it is designed, the importance of reducing inflammation, or how detoxification and lymphatic body work is so magical for our bodies. This lack of information may leave you a little lost.

From personal experience, I will tell you what not to do: Do not try to change everything all at once!

Please for the love of jugs, go slow so you do not get overwhelmed, which will eventually leave you feeling anxious and burnt out.

My story went something like this...

I became a pro in researching 'how to stay cancer free' through books, listening to all the breast cancer podcasts, watching the documentaries, having multiple conversations with different doctors and/or holistic healers, and doing other research to learn as much as I could to stay cancer free. However, I dove in head first and simply tried to change too many things at once.

Over time I became a fear-driven freak about my body. I realized I was going down a path that was not me and not sustainable. I tried switching to a plant-based diet, changed all my beauty and household products, removed as many electromagnetic fields (EMF)s around me as possible, and stopped drinking wine, but all of this led me towards living from a place of desperation rather than joy.

I started to lose my lust for life and felt as if I was turning into a robot, simply going through the motions. My brain was overloaded, and I felt like I was surviving and not thriving. That speed of living was not working for me. Life, in general, is too overwhelming, and if you go at the rate I did in the beginning, it will never last. While yes, I recommend learning as much as you can to create a healthier internal/external environment, you also have to take one day at a time. Please don't do it all at once and, more importantly, have fun with it.

Invite in a sense of levity with trying out new habits and lifestyle changes. Get creative and don't put so much pressure on yourself. As it becomes more natural, then you can start to incorporate others until those become habits and so on and so forth.

It's important to be completely honest with yourself in this process. Take some time to look at your habits, diet, mindset, relationships, etc. Ask yourself:

- What can stay and what needs to go in order to create harmony in my MBHS?
- Where am I self-sabotaging myself?
- What habits create more stress and frustration rather than peace and joy?

If you feel called, write down the answers, then you can use the suggestions below to help shift and create new habits. Again, be real with yourself here and remember we all have habits and characteristics that drain us more than fill us up! It's okay. No one is perfect, and we can all improve in certain areas of our lives.

This is just another opportunity to grow through what you go through and thrive after cancer.

Moral here is I want you to personalize your own growth journey of health and well-being to live an empowered life, not only through but after cancer as well.

Below are more suggestions to add into your repertoire of cancer-fighting habits. I am sure there are hundreds of others, but this should give you a great start.

Remember there is more to your healing and thriving than just your breast. You need to consider your whole self. Some options may seem obvious, and some may prompt you to do your own research to understand the what, why, and how to incorporate it into your lifestyle. Which is exactly my intention.

Think outside the very narrow-minded box of just doctors and medicine. Get curious about the many different types of healing you connect with.

> There is something for everyone, but not everything is for everyone. It's important to understand not every suggestion or practice will align with you, and that's okay.

Pick something (or a few things) that align with you or that you feel could potentially make the biggest impact. Then implement one or two new habits/changes at a time, so you can truly understand the difference it makes in your life. Allow yourself the time to adapt to the changes so they become habits. It takes about sixty-six days to form new habits—ones that stick at that—so go slow in this process.

Just remember regardless of what changes you implement, every little change or shift you make in your life is a step in the right direction towards your ultimate health.

As I have said throughout the book, you have the power of choice! You always get to choose what changes and what stays in your life. Choose wisely.

Below are a few lists of tips and suggestions to get your wheels towards thriving after cancer, not just surviving.

Keep your nervous system in check, reducing stress and creating a positive charge in your mind and energy to regulate your nervous system. It is imperative to reduce as much added stress as possible in your life.

- Meditation
- Journaling
- Intention/Mantra Practice
- Breath-work
- Yoga
- Qigong
- Energy Healing
- EFT Tapping
- Acupressure and/or Acupuncture (which could be in all sections here)
- Gratitude Practice

Create a healthy lymphatic system to remove excess hormones and toxic waste. If you had lymph nodes removed, check with a lymphatic specialist to further assist you.

- Lymph Massage: self or from a specialist

- Rebounding: Basically a mini trampoline. Beneficial and fun!
- Exercise: walking, swimming, weightlifting, yoga. Once again anything; just move your body.
- Dry Brushing
- Castor Oil Packs
- Salt Baths
- Ionic Foot Soaks
- Infrared Sauna

Strengthen your immune system (which directly correlates with your nervous and lymphatic systems as well).

- Get enough sleep
- Add supplements and herbs to your daily routine to strengthen your immunity
- Check on your gut health (Eighty percent of your immune system lives in your gut).
- Reduce inflammation in the body with supplements, food, and weight management)
- Reduce alcohol intake
- IV therapies such as mistletoe

Honor food as medicine.

- Consider plant-based diet
- Buy organic foods: Search for the dirty dozen and clean fifteen for a list of veggies and fruits that are best organic and where you can save.
- Reduce highly processed foods such as cold cuts, hot dogs, packaged foods, and sodas

- Reduce sugar intake. Sugar does not directly feed cancer, according to some sources, but when you consume a lot of artificial sugar, your insulin spikes making your body work overtime to adapt. Daily servings of fruits and veggies with natural sugars are okay.
- Add in organic, non-GMO soy (This may be controversial, but from my research, soy is actually good for estrogen-positive breast cancers).
- Get your cruciferous veggies on: broccoli, cauliflower, brussels sprouts, to name a few.
- Incorporate supplements such as Dim (diindolylmethane), sulforaphane, and/or indole3-carbinol to fight cancer cells. Also good for PMS so win-win. Well, if you still get your period.

Tip about veggies: If you cut and cook your veggies, try this instead. Cut the veggies and let them sit for thirty-five to forty-five minutes before cooking. When cut, there are cancer fighting phytochemicals released, so when you wait to cook them, the phytochemicals are reabsorbed back into the food and remain there when cooking. However, when you cut and cook them right away they burn off with the heat, unfortunately leaving you with a delish veggie but not as strong and potent as they can be.

- Incorporate supplements such as Dim (diindolylmethane), sulforaphane, and/or indole3-carbinol to fight cancer cells. Also good for PMS so win-win. Well, if you still get your period.

Reduce toxins in your environment.

- Reduce exposure to electromagnetic field (EMF): EMFs are everywhere now with cell phones, Bluetooth® devices, computers, tablets, etc. There are many ways to reduce the exposure such as turning off WiFi at night, purchasing EMF blockers for your devices, or wearing EMF blocking jewelry.
- Switch out your beauty products: Find product lines without sulfates, parabens, or fragrance.
- Change your deodorant, removing aluminum and parabens.
- Switch out your household products: Same as your beauty products; your household products should not include harsh chemicals or fragrances.
- Get rid of unsafe cookware. Buy only non-toxic pots and pans with no heavy metals.
- Do not heat up foods or store hot foods in plastic containers. Switch to glass if possible.
- Change your water filtration system in your house to reduce all the chemicals not only for the water you drink but for your showers and sinks too.

Knowledge is power.

- Surround yourself with the "right" people for your journey.
- Hire a functional or naturopathic doctor to create a personalized plan just for you!
- Hire a life coach to help you navigate life after cancer.

- ° Find a local thermographer to add thermography scans to your yearly checkups. Thermography is not a diagnostic tool but a preventive scan to track inflammation in your body.
- ° Listen to health and wellness podcasts or books to learn about how amazing the human body is. There is so much amazing information at your fingertips for free.

Hormone Blockers and Targeted Therapies

This may be a good time to chat about hormone blockers and targeted therapies. Love to love them or love to hate them, but most likely you will be told you need to add hormone blockers or targeted therapy to your cancer journey. This typically follows the completion of chemo, radiation, or surgery. True for most breast cancers, what medication you are recommended will depend on what type of cancer you had and if you are pre- or post-menopausal.

There are a ton of drugs out there currently such as Tamoxifen, Anastrozele, or Letrozole, just to name a few. There seems to be a lot of talk around these types of drugs mainly due to the possible side effects. You will hear things from hot flashes to joint pain or more serious ones like depression, uterine cancer, or osteoporosis. I don't know about you, but none of that sounds fun to me. I doubt you are saying, "Wow, Crissy that sounds amazing, I'm in!"

I giggle saying that, but it's true.

Most doctors will not introduce these as an option, rather it will be a requirement. This is where I think it is really important for you to do your due diligence and take the time to decide if these meds are for you or not. I am not here to persuade you either way, but what I will offer is a voice of reason, reminding you to be your own advocate.

Do your research, ask for more testing to see if your body will react to the drugs in the way they hope, and see what alternatives there are for you. Remember the power of aligned choice. This is the perfect time to tap back into the powers of aligned choice. Make sure whatever you decide is in alignment with your whole self!

Personally, after much contemplation, I opted out. This is my decision and my story only. I do not expect anyone to take the path I chose. Instead, I encourage you to do your own research and listen to your gut to make your own aligned choice.

My decision was not an easy decision. My doctors were definitely not on board and had me second-guessing my decision. Quite honestly, I made a lot of changes to my lifestyle and wanted to take a more natural route in my journey to remain cancer free. Knowing this gave me the power and confidence to kindly decline their recommendation.

Does it mean I will never take medication? No, I will not completely shut the door on Tamoxifen or anything, but for now it does not feel aligned to me. Not to mention, I feel I would probably have gotten every symptom under the sun because I would have been doing it out of fear and not from an aligned place.

I firmly believe that if you are fully on board with taking any medications, specifically in this case hormone blockers or therapies, then your body may receive the medication more gently than if you go into it kicking and screaming! With that said, I know some women who experienced minimal symptoms, but I also met many who were affected big time.

Does it mean you will get every symptom listed on the warning label? No, but quite possibly at the same time! The thing is I do not know how your body will react and here's the kicker, neither do the doctors! No way for anyone to say how your body will react because everyone is different.

None of this is to scare you or even persuade you. This is simply one more opportunity for you to stand in your power, do your own research, and make the aligned choice that is right for you—and not just because your doctors scare you into needing it.

> Your body, your decision, your life.

You get to choose, so choose from an aligned place of harmony within you.

Remember you are worthy of living your best and healthiest life.

Celebrations and Anniversaries

Let's switch gears towards incorporating ways to celebrate life from here on out. I totally understand not everyone likes to celebrate themselves—for whatever reason. It could be because you don't like to be the spotlight, the center of attention, or you may be too busy focusing on others, but I say, "Why the hell not?"

Seriously, you deserve to celebrate your awesomeness any time but especially after cancer.

You have been through so much and, hopefully, appreciate your life even more now. I invite you to go ahead and celebrate life, but I hope you don't need the encouragement from me. I hope you give yourself permission to celebrate, to honor, to live in the present moment.

A goddess thriver, such as yourself, deserves to celebrate so repeat after me, "It is safe to celebrate my awesomeness!"

A thriver understands life is precious. I want you to celebrate the big things, the little things, and everything in between. I wholeheartedly mean this when I say, "You deserve it," and I am so here for it. Like I mentioned earlier in this book, I will be your biggest cheerleader, but you have to be as well.

Celebrate with friends or by yourself—just dedicate time to celebrate everything you have gone through and how far you have come. This transitions beautifully into a discussion about dates that only cancer thrivers will know and appreciate. Cancerversaries, re-birthdays, and other milestone dates.

Cancerversary

No doubt every Pink Sister will remember the exact moment when they heard those words, "You have cancer."

The anniversary of your cancer diagnosis, a day where your life changed in an instant, can be a very heavy time each year. All the more reason why I believe in honoring this day every year.

Both an unforgettable and a certainly powerful day in your life, the date of your diagnosis is considered your cancerversary. For me, my cancerversary brings many emotions to the surface as I remember all the "happenings" around my diagnosis. I use this day as a day of remembrance to process whatever I need to process.

It may not be just one day. For me, I find the days before and after my cancerversary kinda heavy too, because I start remembering where I was and what I did the days following my diagnosis. All bets are off in terms of emotions, and I feel what I need to feel. Sometimes it is sadness, thinking like *Wow, I really can't believe this is my life*, and then sometimes it shifts towards joy when I look at how far I've come. Again, that is my personal experience.

I want you to use this day (or days) however you need to release and process not only emotions but stagnant energy as well that might come to the surface for you. Treat yourself to a day off, a massage, acupuncture, a sunrise, a staycation (or even a big vacation), go to a yoga class, treat yourself to a piece of cake, or spoil yourself with some jewelry. Any and all are amazing.

> For instance, the year I wrote this book I took the day to myself. I watched the sunrise, went to an amazing yoga HiiT (high-intensity interval training) class, followed by acupuncture, a facial, a little writing, and then a yummy, healthy dinner at home with the family. There were tears, screams, laughs...all the feels. It was perfect!

It doesn't have to be anything big; just dedicate time for yourself to move through whatever emotions you need to feel and celebrate your life. You have come a long way and deserve another day to celebrate your amazingness other than your birthday.

Re-birthday

A re-birthday in the cancer world is the day that you receive the news that you are No Evidence of Disease (NED) or cancer free. A re-birthday could either be considered the day your doctor gave you the news, confirming tests and scans to ensure no evidence and margins are clear, or possibly the day of your surgery to remove the cancer. I chose the day of my mastectomy, because I tend to remember that day more than just a phone call telling me the margins were clear and they feel they got it all.

Regardless, I honor my re-birthday by simply taking some time to acknowledge and appreciate this journey. It is not typically a huge celebration for me. I don't really do anything for this day other than taking some time to myself to remember how far I have come. Personally, I tend to celebrate my cancerversary more, but you may be completely different.

I say live it up! This is your life and your journey, so celebrate how you see fit.

As these anniversaries come up, so can lots of emotions. Remember, not every day is all sunshine and rainbows. These anniversaries can and will bring up some heaviness, which is completely normal.

I mention this again because sometimes these anniversaries can be sneaky. Some years may be different than others, so allow yourself to go with the flow because any and all milestones have the potential to bring up lots of memories and emotions. You may think you have released them, but they could still linger so be ready. I think by now you know how I operate and what I am going to say during these times, "Let them up and out!"

I do not want you to suppress any emotions on or around the big dates when it comes to your cancer journey. Find productive ways to release, take the time to drown out the noise, and go inward to see what you need on those days. Yes, again, another perfect time to call in some of your holistic practices to help you in those moments. My favorite go-to healing practices around the time of my anniversaries are meditation, EFT tapping, and jumping into the ocean.

Story Time

Earlier I mentioned what I did for my cancerversary this year, but let me go more into detail. I wanted time by myself so during the car ride to the beach, I allowed myself to scream some profanity and allowed tears to stream down my face.

By the time I got to the beach, I was a little more relaxed, present, and full of appreciation for what was in front of me. Literally and figuratively speaking. I then wrote in my journal, put my feet in the ocean, and found peace in the serene backdrop—all before seven in the morning.

I created the vibe that I wanted (peace), but only after I let myself cry and scream to let go of anger, confusion, sadness, and disappointment. If I held that inside myself, then I truly would not have been able to feel the peace. It would have been a mask that, eventually, would scream to come off.

If you suppress for too long, it can cause other damage so all the more reason to let the emotions up and out as they roll in at any point in your journey. Regardless, do whatever you need to in order to feel the feels.

It boils down to this: Celebrate whatever and however. This should come as no shock; we don't know how long we have on this earth so celebrate. Regardless of *what* milestone you celebrate, just celebrate life.

You deserve to take time to appreciate and honor your life in a meaningful way.

As we wrap up, I pray this book has given you life and inspired you to shine a light amidst the darkness. This is not a goodbye but a **see you later**! Remember, there is no better time than now to thrive in your life. Do not let cancer define you; don't let it take away your essence, or stop you from living the life you deserve.

Other important things to remember are to stay connected to your body, your nervous system, and trust your intuition. Create a life that prioritizes your health, your happiness, your wholeness.

I know this is cliche, but it is so true: You have to fill your cup first, putting on your oxygen mask first before helping others, so love yourself enough to thrive during and after cancer. And always do it in a way that feels aligned to you.

Once again, you are powerful beyond measure, my beautiful *For the Love of Jugs* Breastie. You got this. It has truly been an honor to connect with you during this challenging time in your life. From my heart to yours, thank you for trusting in me.

AFFIRM WITH ME ONE LAST TIME:
I make aligned, present-moment choices that honor my highest self.
I love and trust my intuition will guide me.
I release all fears and step into my power.

**"THE WOUND IS THE PLACE WHERE
THE LIGHT ENTERS YOU." - RUMI**

Be the Light!
ONE LOVE
-Crissy

Breastie's Notes, Thoughts, and Ahas

How can I make choices today that honor my highest self?

When have I trusted my intuition and found it guided me toward what I needed?

How can I release fear and step into my personal power?

Chapter Ten

Reclaim Your Power

I couldn't end this book without one more powerful practice. Included are a few more blank pages for you to write a very special letter to yourself. You can think of this as a letter of agreement, reminding you to step into your power with love, dedication, conviction, and ease. It is also a symbol to break up with cancer's shallow, fear-based mindset.

You have already done so much amazing work to get where you are right now with grace and ease, and this practice is another outlet to release the attachment to cancer. This simple (but not easy) practice is powerful and cathartic but only if you allow yourself to be vulnerable during the process.

First it is really important to set the stage to put yourself in a clear and open-minded space to write the letter.

> ○ Set the tone. Dedicate time where you can be alone (maybe in your zen space) with zero distractions.

- ○ Turn your phone off, light some candles, turn on healing frequency music such as 741Hz, 432 Hz, or 528Hz, and possibly do a meditation before you begin.
- ○ Burn sage or palo santo to create clean energy within you and the space.

Regardless of what you do, the goal is to create a space where you can feel peace with no interruptions. Take the time you deserve to drop in with some breath-work and get grounded. Here we go...

Start the letter like this:

Dear Cancer,
We need to talk. It's not you, it's me. It's time for me to take back my power.

Then write whatever comes up, but please do not over-think this practice. Let your MBHS do the speaking for you, not your brain. Your brain will want to stop you from feeling the emotions but your body needs to release them, so allow yourself to go there! *There* being the place that is full of vulnerability, emotions, and rawness.

This practice is meant to be real, honest, truthful, and I want you to feel it all. Feel it as you write it and write whatever comes up. Don't worry this is not going to be graded by your English teacher, so it doesn't have to make sense to anyone but you. Nor does it have to be in any specific order.

Write as if your future self is writing it. How will she want to feel? What does she want to experience? What will she need to move forward and take back her life? Then create goals to continue moving the needle to a healthier, stronger, happier you. Think big-picture here too with your whole self—Mind, Body, Heart, and Soul (MBHS). This helps ensure you are committed to living a life of joy, good health, and love—on all levels. If you need some inspiration, below are some questions to consider as you write:

- What do I need to release?
- What power am I reclaiming that cancer may have stolen from me?
- What actions will I take moving forward?
- How do I want to feel in my life after cancer?

As you finish, you can either burn it safely or keep it to read if/when you feel a little less than powerful and connected. What you do with it is totally up to you, but I think keeping it rather than burning it is a smart idea.

Why? Mainly because I would be lying if I said thoughts of cancer don't creep up from time to time (even years later), so reading your letter may help you to realign and reset. I have kept mine and read it many times. Sometimes tears of joy come up and sometimes other emotions. All of which is good for your healing but only if you allow yourself to feel them to release them.

This letter is simply one more tool for you to lean into for your healing. If you burn it, let it burn away the negative feelings and vibes as well. If you keep the letter, allow yourself to come back to it anytime you need a little encouragement to live with love and peace rather than fear. One last time, do whatever sets your soul free.

Below is a letter that I wrote to myself.

Dear Cancer,

We need to talk, it's not you it's me...It's time for me to take back my power. I know you needed to express yourself fully in order for me to hear the distress signals that my body was showing. However, I think it is time you go back into hiding. Living these last few months with you has been daunting and tough so I am happy to see you go and get back to my life. I know life will look different now and I am actually ready for it. While you have shown me just how strong I can be and how important my health is, I have decided to make a pact with my wholeness and thrive after you have graced me with your presence. I have decided I am worthy of showing up for myself and will continue to do so every damn day. I will be the most regulated woman the majority of the time unless a bear is chasing me then all bets are off. I will connect to myself daily with meditation, breath-work, movement or other amazing ways to nourish my wholeness. I will use my food as my own medicine cabinet and honor my body. I have judged and shamed it for too long, but today I am ready to lead with love and self compassion and let all other shit go! I deserve my own love. Thank you, Cancer, for showing me how strong I am and leading me to help me tap into my power and my intuition more. I now truly know the answers are within me and I will pause and connect to myself—my WHOLE SELF, more often to stay in Harmony! I hope you understand that I never want to see you again. Sending much love and light.

ONE LOVE,

-Crissy

Now it's time to write your letter. I am holding space for you.

Dear Cancer,

We need to talk, it's not you it's me...It's time for me to take back my power.

Breastie Resources

Books

Anti Cancer: A New Way of Life, David Servan-Schreiber, MD, PhD

Radical Hope, Kelly A. Turner PhD with Tracy White

Breasts: The Owners Manual, Dr. Kristi Funk

Worthy Human, Tracy Litt

Yoga for Cancer, Tari Prinster

How Not to Die, Dr.Michael Greger

Podcasts

Heal with Kelly, Kelly Gores

Chris Beats Cancer, Chris Wark

Born to Heal, Katie Deming

Keeping Abreast With Dr. Jenn Simmons

Dr. Mark Hyman Show, Dr. Mark Hyman

Documentaries

Heal

The C Word

Recipe/CookBooks

The Cancer Kitchen, Rebecca Katz and Mat Edelson
Cooking Through Cancer, Richard Lombardi

List Yours Here

Acknowledgments

This book would not exist without the love, support, and contributions of so many incredible people.

To my husband, Robbie, my rock—your love, patience, and strength have held me through the most challenging moments. From the very beginning—before the diagnosis, through the hardest moments, and even now as I write these words—you have been my unwavering rock. You have stood by my side, cheering me on, lifting me up, and loving me through it all, even on my hardest days when I didn't feel like myself. Thank you for walking beside me on this journey, for the laughter when I needed it most, and for reminding me every day that I am loved. There truly are not enough words to describe my gratitude and love for you. You have shown me what unconditional love looks like, what true partnership means, and what it feels like to be completely seen, supported, and cherished. And clearly, "Thank you" is not enough. But I will say it anyway, with all my heart: Thank you. For everything. Always.

To my children, Gabriel and Antonia, my greatest gifts—your love and light simply inspire me in ways words cannot express. You were the biggest reason I showed up to this diagnosis the way I did. I knew I had to give this fight my everything so I could witness all of the amazing things you will experience and accomplish in your lives. I needed to be an inspiration to you both—to be the example of what determination, peace, strength, love, worthiness, and perseverance look like. Thank you for your endless kindness, resilience, and belief in me. You are my heart walking around outside my body. I hope I made you proud and inspired you to live your lives with the same dedication. Let your light shine so bright that it illuminates not just your own path, but the paths of those around you. Never doubt your strength, your resilience, or the boundless love that surrounds you. You are my greatest joy, my deepest love, and my most precious purpose.

To my family and friends, you know who you are, you are my chosen circle of love—your support has lifted me when I could not stand on my own. There are no words that could ever fully capture the depth of my gratitude for each of you. Between my sisters, sister-in-law, mom, mother-in-law, tons of additional family, and friends, I wish I could name you all but just know you are in my heart. Your love, support, and unwavering presence have been my greatest gifts throughout this journey. You reminded me of my strength when I felt weak, surrounded me with love when I felt uncertain, and cheered me on every step of the way. I am beyond blessed to have such an incredible circle of people who have stood beside me, walked with me, and carried me when I couldn't walk on my own. Thank you! Thank you simply for being there and holding space for me in the hardest moments—you have lifted me in ways I never knew I needed. You are a part of my soul.

To my best friend, Tracy, who nudged and encouraged me to bring this book to fruition. You kept the vision alive in me when doubt crept in, reminding me why this story needed to be told. Your unwavering belief in me, your gentle (and not-so-gentle) pushes, and your endless support have been a gift beyond measure. Thank you for always being in my corner, for knowing when to cheer me on and when to hold space. This book exists, in part, because of you. I am forever grateful for your love, friendship, and light.

To my publishing team, Raven and Jennifer, who helped bring this vision to life—your guidance, patience, and expertise turned my words into a book that I hope will help and heal others. I am beyond grateful for your dedication to this project.

To Michelle Sherman, the brilliant artist behind the illustrations—thank you for capturing the essence of my vision so beautifully. Your work is beyond gorgeous and I am so grateful for your gifts.

To Antonia Rae, my sweet baby girl and gifted photographer. Your talents are forever engraved in my heart and my work. Thank you for capturing my authenticity—the raw, the real, and the beautiful. Your work is a reflection of your kindness and talent, and I could not be more proud of you.

To Jan, Brynn, and Tina, thank you for courageously sharing your stories to help our Pink Sisters feel empowered. Your honesty and strength will inspire and uplift so many on their journey. I am deeply grateful for your trust, support, and the impact we are making together.

And finally, to every person who has walked this path—this book is for you. May you find grace, ease, and the knowing that you are never alone.

This book, this journey, this life—I share it with all of you. Thank you for being my heart, my foundation, and my greatest source of love and light.

From my heart to yours,
ONE LOVE
-Crissy

About the Author

Crissy Florio is a proud mom of two, wife to her high school sweetheart, devoted sister, loving daughter, doting aunt, dog mom, yogi, and friend to many. A breast cancer thriver, Crissy was diagnosed in 2020—a moment that shifted her perspective and led her to embrace a combination of traditional and holistic practices for healing.

By using contemporary medical treatments with the transformative power of her Mind, Body, Heart, and Soul (MBHS), Crissy cultivated a path of grace and resilience through one of life's greatest challenges. Her journey is a testament to the healing power of inner calm and connection, even in the face of a cancer diagnosis.

Today, Crissy uses her experience to inspire and empower others affected by cancer to live with purpose, connection, and peace. Through workshops, speaking engagements, yoga classes, and her writing, she helps others tap into their inner strength, foster positive energy, and reclaim a life of thriving—not just surviving.

Crissy's mission is to help others unlock their MBHS potential, proving that healing is not just about survival, it's about rediscovering the joy, beauty, and power within.

Connect with Crissy at www.fortheloveofjugs.com and on Instagram @Flo_withCrissyFlorio or her website www.healinginharmony.net.

www.ingramcontent.com/pod-product-compliance
Lightning Source LLC
Chambersburg PA
CBHW021138130626
46554CB00005B/1569